How to Sur[vive]
on a
Toxic Planet

Dr. Steve Nugent

Second Edition printing

Published by *The Alethia Corporation*

To order additional copies of this book, please contact: Dupli-Pack at 1-888-443-1979 or visit: **www.glycotools.com**

The information in this book is not intended or recommended as a means of diagnosing or treating any physical or mental condition. All matters concerning physical and mental health should be supervised by a health practitioner knowledgeable in treating that particular condition.

Dedication:

This book is about the environment and your health, so I want to dedicate this book to many people. I would like to first thank all doctors of every discipline and from every school who are open-minded and willing to look at complementary medicine as part of the solution to the problems we have in health care today. It takes courage to step outside the box! They are special people who are willing to take criticism and sometimes even put their careers at risk by using modalities that are not yet accepted by the mainstream. It takes a person with unique inner strength and a selfless desire to serve the needs of others. It also takes a very secure person to admit that he or she doesn't know everything and then be receptive to new ideas.

I especially salute the naturopaths of all schools and philosophies for their courage to fight the "old school" way of doing things. Theirs has not been an easy path, and still isn't. I know that more than anyone!

I need to thank my beautiful wife, Wendy, for giving up many of our years together while I was off doing research, teaching and working a practice that had a never-ending supply of patients in need. My family was always patient as I spent a great deal of time away from them, flying around the world to fight for the rights of all complementary medicine practitioners. I was ridiculed and scorned by people who did not know the truth or would not listen to the truth. Although Wendy spent many lonely weeks and months without me, her support for me never wavered.

I must also thank my son who spent much of his childhood without my involvement. Please forgive me, son. I think the sacrifice will pay off for all the children of this world who will benefit from my mission. My family has always supported my tireless crusade. They know the answers must be found before it is too late. We must heal ourselves and the planet. We all know the alterative.

I want to thank everyone who has believed in my quest and has not only stood by me through personal attacks but has walked beside me on the side of truth. We must unite and work together so that we may survive a world that we have made toxic.

So I dedicate this book to everyone who has the vision, the courage and the heart to make sacrifies necessary to save life on this planet.

Someone I respect very much once said to me, "If you are being attacked, then you must be doing something right." Thank you, Sam, for your support and encouragement.

Steve Nugent, NMD, PhD

Contents

Contents

Why this book?

I have been lecturing on the issues addressed in this book for many years, but I have never before sat down to put all of this information under one cover. Much of this is information that the government, industry and media have not (for various reasons) communicated to you. These facts should play a major role in your decision-making process for your health as well as the health of those you love. It should also be key for making decisions on Election Day. You need to know how to make your home and workplace as safe and healthy as possible. Without this information you cannot make intelligent, well-informed decisions.

Over the years, I wrote many articles on health in my international newsletter, which was read by doctors and laymen in 17 countries, and before the popularity of the Internet, I made a minor impact. Through 11 years of many TV and radio guest appearances, I've reached millions. However, too many of those listeners or viewers would stay motivated on these issues for only hours or days. Apathy and distractions happen all too easily. It is normal for most people to assume someone else will take care of the problem and indeed that government will take care of them as well, and that there is no personal responsibility or effort required on their part.

Many books have been published, such as Rachel Carson's **Silent Spring**, which was probably the most important book of its type, since it broke new ground for environmental awareness. Many other excellent books, such as **The Truth About Where You Live** and **Our Stolen Future**, also gave me hope that the media would catch on and inform the public, which would then force government and industry by the power of their votes and dollars to take the actions that had to be taken to save our planet and the human race. However, this has not happened. Clearly, this information will only have impact if it is in print. However, unless the facts presented here are read, embraced and acted upon by hundreds of thousands, the movement toward saving the world will not be successful.

This book is my attempt to reach anyone who will listen. Time is of the essence. Our species (and every species!) on this planet is in imminent danger. Greed, selfishness, sloth, apathy and ignorance have created an environment that is now manifesting itself in disease, suffering and death in our populations. There is still time and there is still hope if we do the right things and take the right actions. But the window of opportunity is closing fast. If we continue on our present course of polluting our planet and ourselves and do not take appropriate action for our personal health as well as the health of our world, this beautiful blue planet will become just another barren, uninhabited rock in space.

History is full of lessons of people who did not heed warnings and as a result perished without hope. Noah tried to warn the people of the impending deluge, and Lot tried to warn the people of Sodom and Gomorrah, but to no avail. Humans have always acted only when forced to act–at the last moment, when a coming catastrophe became undeniably obvious. Yet most often, when people finally took action, it was too late to avoid the consequences of their hesitation.

In this book, I will pull no punches. I will also use "truth tactics" that may be labeled "scare tactics" by some, but I must do everything I can to urge you to take action before it is too late.

I cannot accomplish this mission alone. I know in my heart that now is the time when many hundreds of thousands of people that I have had the honor to teach are now ready to embark on a mission for world health. Not just a mission for the health of the world's people, but for the Earth itself. These hundreds of thousands of caring, wonderful people can become millions, who in turn will become tens of millions. It is only through our efforts together that we can save our planet from ultimate oblivion.

This book will be your first guidebook on the true, scientifically confirmed dangers in the environment with solutions for your health and the health of our world. These are dangers you may not be able to see, taste or smell, but that cause needless suffering, disease and death. Our planet does not have to die, and our children should not have to suffer in a toxic world. We can prevent birth defects and disease in the majority of cases. We do not need to see species after species disappear and pass into history. We do not have to cope with an ever-increasing level of degenerative diseases along with all the suffering that goes with them, both for the victims and their families. We can make a difference, but we must act now! We must act with logic and objectivity and not wait until some government official explains why the proper procedure will take x number of years.

This book, unlike other good books I have mentioned, will deal with the environment and our personal health. However, it will also discuss why the old thought processes are still being taught at medical schools and in university nutrition science departments–obsolete thought processes that are still embraced by government officials even though they are no longer valid. Finally, this book will provide you with the recommendations and education you need to embark on a course of health for yourself, your loved ones and your planet.

There is still time to act, but the clock keeps ticking...

How to Survive on a Toxic Planet

on a

Toxic Planet

SECTION 1

Understanding
the Problem

Dr. Steve Nugent

Chapter 1
What set me on this course?

Back in 1977, I began educating the public about dietary supplements and dietary deficiencies. I naively thought I would someday have a thriving practice based on preventive health and education. I dreamed of a large preventive health clinic, research and teaching center where I would educate patients and doctors alike.

But that's not exactly how it worked out.

It took many years of hard work and study. Eventually I had the clinic of my dreams, at least in terms of brick and mortar. My clinic in Michigan had a large classroom area next to the lab, where I conducted free classes on proper eating habits, dietary supplements and exercise. My hope was that by educating people, they would take the right steps for their health to prevent the onset of illness or disease. I tried hard to attract those who were symptom-free in order to educate them on preventives. However, that was not to be.

After having success with supposedly "hopeless" cases, my reputation began to spread. In fact, many of my colleagues referred to my clinic as "the last chance clinic." I had patients coming from every continent, often accompanied by translators.

Although I was dedicated to my patients, I was poorly suited psychologically for that sort of patient load. Every night in my mind, I took all of my patients home with me. I refused to give up on those who had given up on themselves. My wife commented that we may as well put a bed and shower in the clinic since I would work very late, frequently falling asleep at my desk only to awaken in the early morning hours.

Early on, I was struck by the fact that the human body is actually an organic machine, requiring specific organic fuels so that it can accomplish the truly miraculous tasks it is designed to perform. The human body is not designed to eat synthetic substances, nor can it heal or cure itself with synthetic fuels. Brain and body chemicals are natural in origin. The most logical way to assist the body in healing itself is through the appropriate natural fuels. This means vitamins, minerals, amino acids, essential fatty acids, phytochemicals (healthful plant chemicals) and the newest category of supplements—glyconutrients–that I will discuss in Chapter 9.

During my relentless search for answers, I tested more than 6,000 dietary supplements of every category and type. It took many years, and I found the majority had no value that we could document by conventional tests, such as changes in blood or urine. I was disappointed more than 85% of the time. Of the thousands of brands on the market I found only about twenty brands that were efficacious, and I used products from those companies, but relied heavily on only two. The fabulous claims the companies made were, for the most part, all talk. Slick advertising was disguised as science. It's no wonder that medical doctors in general have such poor opinions of dietary supplements. Most so-called supplements are indeed worthless. (Note: I will discuss the latest scientifically validated supplements in "The Solution" section of this book, which offers some specific recommendations for surviving on our toxic planet.)

The psychological conditioning that accompanies training in Western biomedicine is that if you have no symptom, you are well. If a symptom does develop, then you seek traditional allopathic medical treatment, such as drugs or surgery. Indeed, the popular rule of thumb in the 20th century was to "eat right, exercise, and you won't get sick." Eating right is extremely important, and exercise is also vital to good health. But those two considerations alone simply are not sufficient to achieve and maintain optimal health in the 21st century.

Right now there are still many dubious "experts" in diet, nutrition and health care who will tell you that dietary supplements are simply not necessary. They proclaim in their books and during talk show appearances, "Eat right, and you won't get sick." Unfortunately, many of these so-called experts simply are not current on the true extent of the threats to human health that exist on this planet today. They are not informed or up-to-date on how little nutrition is actually being delivered to us in our food.

However, if they read this book, they will be!

I will answer a number of questions in this book that can be grouped in four major areas:

1. What is the full extent of the current threats to your health?

2. What role do toxins play in disease and illness?

3. What are the threats that exist in your home and work place?

4. What are safe, non-toxic alternatives to these threats?

I will not close, however, without providing tips and recommendations to help you and your family cope with the inescapable threats that exist, in addition to what we can do to improve our planet's condition. Always remember as you are reading this book that there is hope, and the Solution Section of the book will offer suggestions and solutions for many of the issues I have written about. So don't get discouraged and don't give up. You'll be amazed to find out what you personally can do for yourself and the planet.

Chapter 2
More Stress, But Less Fuel

Before discussing solutions that can help keep you healthy, I want to help you understand the magnitude of the problems. Let's deal first with the concept of stress. Everyone has heard that stress kills. Most people think that means psychological stress. But there are a number of different types of stress that affect your health and may contribute to illness, disease and even premature death.

• Psychological Stress
Scientific studies have clearly shown that psychological stress does, in fact, lower immune function.[1-5] As you read this book, you will learn that anything that could lower your immune function is dangerous to you in the 21st century. We now know that even having negative thoughts can lower your immune function. Do you know anyone who can get through a day without having a single negative thought?

The more stress, the greater the demand for organic fuel just to maintain an even playing field. Illness, such as fibromyalgia, reinforces that theory.[6-9] The onset of fibromyalgia can nearly always be correlated with a marked increase in psychological or physical stress, a stressful event or trauma. Indeed, in those cases where the disorder seems to have been banished from the patient's life, increased psychological stress can often bring it roaring back.

• Physical Stress
Many people are unaware of what their body was actually designed to do. This amazing organic machine we live in was, in fact, designed to defend itself, heal itself and protect itself from all manner of threats. However, the human body was also designed to live on a planet that no longer exists.

When our earliest ancestors began walking the earth, the world was a pristine place. Psychological stress was extremely low, and environmental stress was non-existent. Physical stress was proportionate to what the body was capable of doing.

As the body creates energy to move our muscles, we release tiny molecules called free radicals. Free radicals—as long as they are controlled by antioxidants—cause no damage to the body. That's because the human body was designed to cope with a normal amount of free radical release during energy production, using antioxidants that come from fruits and vegetables as well as chemicals made in the body, such as glutathione.

We no longer live in the world we were designed to live in. The environmental and dietary stresses that we now have create a situation where our body's normal mechanisms for creating glutathione and utilizing antioxidants from foods are inadequate to protect us from these stresses. This results in fatigue, lethargy, lack of clarity of thought, illness, disease and premature death. **The more stress, the greater the demand for organic fuel just to maintain an even playing field.**

• Dietary Stress
The human body was designed to function perfectly with a good, fresh, raw, natural diet. Originally, there were no processed, refined or prepackaged foods. There were no grocery stores. Individuals had to hunt and/or gather what they ate. Foods were the freshest and most nutritious that have ever existed on this planet. There were no cupcake or biscuit bushes. No white bread trees. You couldn't pull French fries out of the

ground. Fruits and vegetables didn't come canned, cooked, dried or packed in refined sugar syrup. Unlike today, people worked hard physically to earn their food. All we have to do now is coast up to the drive-through window, or walk a few paces to the refrigerator.

Our bodies were, in fact, designed to earn our food.

Food should be fresh, raw and natural. We should eat raw food whenever appropriate, yet very few people do so these days. We are conditioned to crave and enjoy foods that have been heated. Food that has been processed with heat in any form loses nutrition. Some heated foods become nothing but empty calories. These foods contribute to adverse insulin reactions that can eventually result in diabetes, a disease that is growing so rapidly that the World Health Organization says it will soon reach epidemic proportions. Some heated and other processed foods also contribute to heart disease and cancers, as well as obesity.

• Environmental Stress
Without a doubt, environmental stress is the most serious threat to human health in the 21st century.

First, let's dispel the myth that diet is sufficient to maintain good health any more. The bar chart labeled "Comparison between Primitive and Modern Man's Intake of Some Vitamins, Minerals and Fiber" (Plate 1, found in the center section of the book) compares what hunter-gatherers consumed nutritionally in their fresh, raw and natural diet with the modern required daily allowance (RDA).[10] What's interesting is the required daily allowance is thought by many people to be the absolute maximum amount that you could possibly consume. That was once true, but it is now simply no longer the case. The required daily allowance varies from country to country. But in most countries—especially the USA—it is the bare minimum amount required to maintain any semblance of health and to keep you from getting a nutritional deficiency disease. The yellow bars on this chart indicate very clearly the very wide gap between being truly healthy and being barely healthy, which means being susceptible to a nutritional deficiency disease.

In 1941, the National Academy of Sciences in the United States became the first agency to establish a required minimum amount of vitamins and minerals. They did so because they were concerned about school children not receiving the minimum nutritional input to keep from acquiring a deficiency disease. Despite the fact that food was plentiful in the United States, nutritional deficiency diseases such as pellagra and beriberi were still being reported since volume and calories are not necessarily synonymous with nutrition and good health.

Nutritional deficiency diseases are not a thing of the past. Even where calories are plentiful in modern nations, these diseases still occur. Scurvy, a disease caused by lack of vitamin C, was virtually eliminated, thanks to the work of Scottish physician James Lind in 1795. He showed that eating small amounts of fresh, natural fruit containing vitamin C would prevent the disease. However, in the 1990s, scurvy was again being documented in modern nations where there were adequate food supplies because of the disproportionate consumption of refined, empty foods.[11]

Beriberi is a disease caused by a deficiency in thiamine (vitamin B_1). Although the cause of beriberi was discovered more than a century ago in the 1890s, it is still being documented in nations where there is plenty of food. Alcohol lowers B_1 with every drink, which by the way contributes significantly to hangovers. Eating refined foods like polished white rice provides no B_1 because the B_1 is in the brown outer husk of the rice.

Ironically, most governments now require that synthetic B_1 be added back after refining brown natural grains into white, worthless grains.

B_1 is what is called a "stress vitamin" since psychological stress reduces B_1, as will illness and immune stress. In diabetic and cancer patients, B_1 deficiencies can become serious enough to bring on beriberi. **Once again, more stress means your body requires more organic fuel just to stay even.**

Pellagra is a disease caused by a deficiency of niacin (vitamin B_3). A severe deficiency of B_3 can lead to the four D's—dermatitis, diarrhea, dementia and death. Although most people think pellagra has been eliminated in modern nations, it hasn't. It is still documented in those who are tryptophan- (an amino acid) deficient as well as in alcoholics and those using certain pharmaceutical drugs.[12]

Pellagra is typically seen only in those whose diet lacks proteins, particularly if their diet is principally corn. It also sometimes occurs in people with gastrointestinal diseases that result in poor absorption of vitamins.

At the beginning, pellagra is characterized by weakness, insomnia and weight loss. Dermatitis follows and is typically worse on skin exposed to sunlight. The skin becomes rough, reddened and scaly. Very painful mouth lesions develop at the same time or soon after. The patient experiences loss of appetite, indigestion and diarrhea. As the disease progresses, the nervous system becomes involved, and includes symptoms such as headache, vertigo, generalized aches, muscular tremors and mental disturbances.

Successful treatment includes the administration of B_3 and the other B-complex vitamin supplements, as well as the addition of natural proteins and fresh vegetables. Protein foods successfully used include milk, lean meat or fish and whole grain cereals (other than corn). B_3 is also considered a stress vitamin. **Again, the more stress, the more organic fuel is needed just to stay even.**

Another nutritional deficiency disease being documented today is called megaloblastic anemia. It is also known as pernicious anemia, or simply B_{12} anemia. Prior to 1926, this form of anemia was actually fatal to about one percent of the population.[12]

This particular nutritional deficiency disease is caused by a deficiency of vitamin B_{12} and folic acid, which causes the bone marrow to produce red cells that are larger than normal, but with reduced oxygen-carrying ability although vitamin B_{12} is the principal deficiency. Without its synergist, folic acid (folate), it is difficult to resolve the problem. It is most common in people over 40 because our ability to digest foods and absorb nutrients such as B_{12} efficiently declines after that age and continues to worsen as we get older. The disease is therefore more often caused by decreased B_{12} absorption rather than by a deficient diet.

Fatigue is the principal and most common symptom of this anemia, but other symptoms include pallor (paleness of the skin not due to genetics), shortness of breath, dizziness and digestive disorders. Inadequately informed vegetarians may suffer from mild to serious B_{12} anemia and its symptoms. It may also be seen in hyperthyroidism and pregnancy. Poor diet is a definite cause, and certain medical treatments, such as IF chemotherapy drugs, may induce it as well.[12]

At the present time, deficiencies of 11 macro minerals, as well as several trace elements, are still being documented. Individuals who suffer from inflammatory bowel diseases (IBDs), diabetes malabsorption, cirrhosis and alcoholism are often deficient in minerals.[12] IBDs (Crohn's disease and ulcerative colitis) affect as many as two million people each year in the United States alone.

In addition, inadequate soil content is often a cause. The resulting disorder is called pica, where typically pregnant women, but also some others who are hugely mineral-deficient, actually eat dirt.[12]

Pica is a disorder in which the patient is so starved for minerals that they continually crave non-nutritive substances such as plaster, paint, paper, dirt, string, wood, crayons and cloth. This odd behavior does not typically interfere with eating normal foods however. (The word pica, in case you are interested, comes from the Latin word for magpie. The ancient Romans believed that magpies ate only earth and clay because they always observed them pecking at the ground.)

In parts of the southeastern United States, the eating of clay by pregnant women and adolescent girls has traditionally been considered healthy and is still often done in that region. When this cultural factor can be verifiably traced as the cause of this behavior in any individual, it is not pica but rather a cultural behavior.

While a definite connection is arguable between mineral deficiencies and mental retardation, pica is sometimes observed among the mentally retarded or those who are developmentally disabled. It has also been observed in children who are emotionally deprived or neglected.

Vitamin D deficiencies historically related to rickets and osteomalacia are still being documented. Insufficient diet or reduced sun exposure have been the historical causes of these diseases, but our diets today have strayed far from our intended natural diets— so far, in fact, that the deficiency can be found even in some people who consume adequate calories.

Unsupplemented dairy products can actually cause vitamin D deficiency. Calcium requires vitamin D to be utilized, and calcium is a dominant molecule over both vitamin D and magnesium. Taking in more calcium or calcium food sources than you have vitamin D to balance it will result in a deficiency of vitamin D. Malabsorption, cholestasis (a slowing or stopping of bile from the gall bladder), IBD and fat-blocking drugs can also lead to vitamin D deficiency.[12]

Deficiencies of vitamin A are commonly linked to poor diet. This deficiency is most commonly observed among urban poor, the elderly and alcoholics.[12]

Studies done in the 1990s are, for the most part, the broadest ever done. But common sense tells us that our eating habits and food sources are not improving. Calories and nutrients are not necessarily synonymous.

It is also extremely important to note that nutritional deficiencies rarely occur in isolation. Everything in nutritional biochemistry is inter-linked. It is difficult (though not impossible) to be deficient in just one factor. The issue isn't that there aren't more nutritional deficiency problems, but rather that sufficient testing and education in this area is unavailable to most physicians. Medical doctors (MDs) and even osteopaths (DOs) are trained in drugs and surgery. The training they do get (if any) in nutrition is not only too brief but typically out-of-date diet and nutritional information as it relates to both prevention and treatment of disease. This should be clear to any physician reading this book. This is the fault of the educational system, so don't blame your physician.

As a side note, I am always amazed when a patient asks his or her doctor if a dietary supplement is alright to take. MDs, with very rare exceptions, do not have adequate training in the therapeutic use of dietary supplements. They often know less factual information than some of the general public. I am never surprised when a doctor, who has no clue what a dietary supplement really is or does, tells his or her patient not to take the supplement or says it could be harmful. It's like asking a plumber how to fix your roof. Before wasting time asking a doctor for advice in matters about which they may not be well-informed, ask about your MDs or DOs level of training in natural supplements.

Medical doctors are taught objectivity, but for some of them, this objectivity seems to be selective. MDs are people—exceptional people, but people nonetheless. They cannot be expected to know absolutely everything that relates to health, although some rare MDs do take additional training in natural therapies. NDs (doctors of naturopathy) or NMDs (doctors of naturopathic medicine) are trained specifically in the therapeutic use of dietary supplements, as well as in all the other natural therapies. Some NDs and NMDs have both allopathic (medical) and naturopathic training, and others do not. All naturopaths have training in the use of dietary supplements, but their levels of knowledge can differ considerably.

Some (but, alas, not all!) chiropractic doctors are trained in the use of natural therapeutics, but only on a limited basis in line with their health philosophies. Yet chiropractors recommend more dietary supplements than any other doctors except NDs and NMDs!

Among Americans over 50, for instance, 65% surveyed say dietary supplements are a necessity[13], and more medical schools are beginning to realize that the public demands increased use of natural therapies. To that end, more courses in integrative, complementary and alternative medicine are being taught in medical schools. MDs who can talk nutrition are in demand and fast becoming prosperous, even famous, while most NDs and NMDs still struggle to make a living. I find that ironic, to say the least.

The ideal doctor of the future will understand both allopathic and naturopathic medicine. I hope naturopathy survives and allopathic medicine converts. Only time will tell.

Now, let's return to the realities of dietary stress. It was in 1989 that the National Academy of Sciences (NAS) did a full and complete re-evaluation of all vitamins and minerals and their requirements.[14] In 1995, the United States Department of Agriculture (USDA) recommended that adults consume 5-9 servings of antioxidant-rich fruits and vegetables each day.[15]

Antioxidants are substances that can neutralize free radicals and render them harmless. Free radicals not neutralized by antioxidants cause damage to your cells and, if left unchecked, can cause free radical oxidative stress diseases, including cancer and heart disease. They also contribute to other illnesses such as diabetes, as well as the aging process itself.[16,17]

The USDA told us that we should eat two to four servings of fruit and three to five servings of vegetables every day in order to get the minimum antioxidant support we need from our food. However, five to nine servings daily of fresh raw fruits and vegetables wasn't terribly realistic, and, of course, almost no one followed these recommendations. They were not only inconvenient, but the majority of Americans simply didn't want to eat that much healthy food each day. Even if they wanted to, it simply wasn't economically feasible for millions of Americans.

Too often, refined food packages, with so-called nutrition facts labeled on the package, lead people to think that they are getting more nutrition than they actually are. Our system of medicine has also conditioned people to think that as long as they are symptom-free, they are well. Since many people have no obvious symptoms and believe they get adequate nutrition from refined foods, there has been no motivation to eat fresh fruits and vegetables at the levels recommended by USDA or NAS.

In the year 2000, the National Academy of Sciences evaluated only those nutrients that are known to be either antioxidants or catalysts for antioxidants.[17] The statement subsequently issued by NAS said that Americans were getting approximately 50% lower levels of certain antioxidants (e.g., vitamin A) from their food than had been previously estimated. NAS did not advocate any specific dietary supplement but recommended that Americans simply double their intake of fruits and vegetables. The comparison of USDA nutrient estimates and actual measurements on page (?) reinforce this point. The actual amount of nutrition as compared to estimates is as much as 28% in some foods, and almost no one realizes that much of the information from USDA is educated guesswork, not actual fact.

Even if you wanted to become a cow grazing all day long on your 18 servings, could you afford to do that? Would you even have the time to graze all day long? You'd spend so much time eating that there would be no time remaining for anything else. Later in this book you will learn that foods have become so deficient since the 1950s that some natural foods have to be consumed at more than 25 times the previous levels to get the same nutrition we got back in the 1950s. The foods may look the same, but the similarity ends there. Remember: Calories will keep you going, but only complete nutrition will keep the body healthy.

All medical and healthcare practitioners at every level are taught that we should be able to get our basic nutrition from food. This premise is based on outdated information that does not take into account the full spectrum of the threats and stresses to human health in the 21st century. I want all people to eat right, consuming fresh, raw and natural foods as much as possible. Realistically, we know most people will not do so. But if they do not, their health will be compromised without essential nutritional support from scientifically validated dietary supplements.

Right now, the only thing that makes sense is to use dietary supplements to provide adequate antioxidant protection. Not all dietary supplements are created equal. I will discuss dietary supplements more specifically in "The Solution" section of this book.

> **"Only 1% of the US population consumes a diet meeting the five food group recommendations that are the basis for the food pyramid in the Dietary Guidelines for America."**
>
> *–American Journal of Clinical Nutrition*, 1997[18]

Even the *Journal of the American Medical Association* (JAMA) has finally entered the modern age by publishing an article that stated, "Most people do not consume an optimal amount of all vitamins by diet alone . . . It appears prudent for all adults to take vitamin supplements."[19]

That JAMA article was a huge step forward for medical doctors everywhere. There can be no doubt that dietary supplements are no longer a luxury. In the 21st century they are a necessity!

Dietary supplements need to be in everyone's monthly budget just as you budget for food, fuel for your car, water, and all of the other daily necessities. In a separate chapter, I'll discuss all of the categories of dietary supplements necessary to achieve and maintain optimal health. I will also discuss dietary supplements probably unknown to most readers of this book. Then I will cover the latest scientific, fully objective data on how these nutrients can not only help you maintain optimal health, but how many of them have actually assisted the body against some of the most serious diseases and illnesses known.

You may be surprised to find out what these nutrients are and just what they can do for you!

References

1. DeKeyser F. Psychoneuroimmunology in critically ill patients. *AACN Clinical Issues.* 2003;14(1):25-32.
2. Schedlowski M, Schmidt RE. [Stress and the immune system]. *Naturwissenschaften.* 1996;83(5):214-220.
3. Adams DO. Molecular biology of macrophage activation: a pathway whereby psychosocial factors can potentially affect health. *Psychosom Med.* 1994;56(4):316-327.
4. Fricchione GL, Bilfinger TV, Hartman A, et al. Neuroimmunologic implications in coronary artery disease. *Adv Neuroimmunol.* 1996;6(2):131-142.
5. Fricchione G, Daly R, Rogers MP, Stefano GB. Neuroimmunologic influences in neuropsychiatric and psychophysiologic disorders. *Acta Pharmacol Sin.* 2001 Jul;22(7):577-587.
6. Bigatti SM, Cronan TA. An examination of the physical health, health care use, and psychological well-being of spouses of people with fibromyalgia syndrome. *Health Psychol.* 2002;21(2):157-166.
7. Cohen H, Neumann L, Shore M, Am et al. Autonomic dysfunction in patients with fibromyalgia: application of power spectral analysis of heart rate variability. *Semin Arthritis Rheum.* 2000;29(4):217-227.
8. Anthony KK, Schanberg LE. Juvenile primary fibromyalgia syndrome. *Curr Rheumatol Rep.* 2001;3(2):165-171.
9. Amir M, Kaplan Z, Neumann L, et al. Post-traumatic stress disorder, tenderness and fibromyalgia. *J Psychosom Res.* 1997;42(6):607-613.
10. Ramberg J, McAnalley BH. From the farm to the kitchen table: a review of the nutrient losses in foods. *GlycoScience & Nutrition.* 2002;3(5):1-12.
11. Prinzo ZW. Scurvy and its prevention and control in major emergencies. WHO/NHD/99.11,World Health Organization: 1999.
12. *Cecil Textbook of Medicine.* W. B. Saunders Company; Philadelphia, PA.,1992.
13. Nutrition Business Journal, 2001 Consumer Research, 1999-2001 http://www.nutritionbusiness.com/data.htm
14. National Academy of Sciences. *Diet and Health.* Washington, D.C.: National Academy Press, 1989.
15. Nutrition and Your Health: Dietary Guidelines for Americans. Home and Garden Bulletin No. 232, USDA and USDHHS, 1995.
16. McAnalley BH, Vennum E, Ramberg J, et al. Antioxidants: consolidated review of potential benefits. *GlycoScience & Nutrition.* 2004;5(1):1-21.
17. Packer L, Colman C. *The Antioxidant Miracle.* John Wiley & Sons, Inc. New York, 1999.
18. Panel of Micronutrients. Dietary reference intakes for vitamin A, vitamin K, arsenic, boron, chromium, copper, iodine, iron, manganese, molybdenum, nickel, silicon,

vanadium, and zinc. Food and Nutrition Board, 2001.

19. Krebs-Smith SM, Cleveland LE, Ballard-Barbash R, et al. Characterizing food intake patterns of American adults. *Am J Clin Nutr.* 1997;65(4 Suppl):1264S-1268S.

20. Fletcher RH, Fairfield KM. Vitamins for chronic disease prevention in adults: clinical applications. *JAMA.* 2002;287(23):3127-3129.

Chapter 3
Oxidative Stress–The Greatest Threat to Your Health

The newest and most serious threat to human health is called oxidative stress. We have already spoken briefly about free radicals. When these free radicals exceed what your body can cope with, they cause damage to your cells, and even to your DNA. In fact, many people are being diagnosed with genetic diseases who might not have a genetic disease at all, but rather have damaged DNA–the result of certain types of free radicals, such as the hydroxyl radical.

Disease Processes Associated with Increased Oxidative Stress[1]

AIDS	Inflammatory bowel disease
Adult respiratory distress syndrome	Myocardial ischemia
Adolescent seizures	Myositis
Alzheimer's disease	Nephritis
Amylotrophic lateral sclerosis (ALS)	Parkinson's disease
Cancer	Pre-eclampsia
Cataracts	Retinopathy
Cerebral vascular accident	Respiratory distress syndrome of neonates
Chronic renal failure	Rheumatoid arthritis
Crohn's disease	Scleroderma
Diabetes mellitus	Sepsis
Hematological disorders	Systemic lupus erythematosus
Hepatitis	Transplantations
Hypertension	Ulcerative colitis
Hypoxia	

In the early 1980s, I modified my lectures, moving from my more optimistic talks that were intended to simply educate people on the proper diet and dietary supplements for good health. I began to introduce information—very often shocking information—about the threats to human health from the environment. Much of what I was lecturing on in the '80s was based on correlation. Studies were not available to verify much of what I believed to be true based on clinical observation. Occasionally, I would share my personal theories with the audience. Very often I received more than a little ridicule from my critics.

One of my theories was that the increase in Parkinson's disease was not necessarily due to genetic factors. There seemed to be a correlation between toxins and concentrations of individuals with Parkinson's.

From Ridicule to Validation
I have been ridiculed for my theories for as long as I can remember. However some of them have become self-evident over time and frankly I really don't care who thinks they came up with it before me. All scientists should be working together for the betterment of life on this planet. Although I have come up with many theories that have since proven out, I do not have the resources to follow through with studies, and not all of my theo-

ries have turned out to be correct. One example is when I first publicly discussed my theory about toxins and Parkinson's in a public lecture at the University of California at Los Angeles in 1997. I was ridiculed, but it didn't take long to get some validation for my theory. Before beginning my lecture day in LA about year later, I opened up *The Los Angeles Times* and saw an article in which scientists said that it was their belief that toxins were causing Parkinson's in most cases, not genetics. Apparently there were scientists who did believe as I did and had the funds to research this. I applaud these courageous scientists because they too no doubt were ridiculed. Recent research has continued to validate this theory.[2,3] With the meager resources I have for research, I have to rely on correlations to lead me in a particular direction, but I am always very pleased to see solid university study validate my correlations and theories. How many people heard that new point of view? How many doctors heard it?

Several years ago, the famous actor, Michael J. Fox, whom we have all enjoyed so much over the years, was diagnosed with Parkinson's. He absolutely does not fit the parameters of someone with Parkinson's disease, according to the medical texts. He is much too young, has no genetic history, etc. Mr. Fox is one famous example, but I believe that over the next few decades we will see many diseases being directly linked to toxins in the environment.

> **"In most cases Parkinson's disease is tied to environment, not just genes, researchers say."**
> *–Los Angeles Times*, 1/27/99

"Seventy-three Percent of All Premature Death Is Due To Oxidative Stress"[4]

Dr. Les Packer of the University of California at Berkeley is one of the world's leading experts in antioxidants–so much so that his colleagues refer to him as "Dr. Antioxidant." He states that 73% of <u>all</u> premature death is due to oxidative stress. Seventy-three percent of all premature death! **Imagine the impact that we could have, not only on your life and the lives of those you love, but also on lives around the planet if we could simply make people understand that antioxidant protection is absolutely essential in today's world.** We must give those people objective, scientific data about which antioxidants would be the most useful for their health. As you will learn in a later chapter, there are many products being sold as antioxidants that either have no antioxidant effect, poor antioxidant effect and/or even a pro-oxidative effect. In other words, some products being sold as antioxidants will actually harm your body. But we will cover all of this in a later chapter.

Keep Your Immune System Ready!

It's often a shock to the average person to learn that every human being makes cancer cells every day. It's not a question of if you will make cancer cells. The relevant questions are: What will your body do when you produce cancer cells? Will your body be able to cope with this challenge? Can your immune system rise to the occasion?

Clearly, at least one out of every three Americans will get cancer[5]–and the statistics are the same or similar in nearly every modern nation that has reported statistics to the World Health Organization (WHO). Cancer victims' bodies are not able to cope with this threat. They are not up to the challenge.

Cancer is an insidious disease. It takes years for cancer cells to reach the point where they can be diagnosed. In breast cancer, for example, it takes an average of five to 30 years for cancer cells to grow and accumulate before cancer can be diagnosed. Every day of every year that the cancer grows in your body, you still feel fine. You have no symptoms, and there are no signs or warnings. Not everyone can go by genetics alone.

Being symptom-free doesn't mean you are well. It simply means you have no obvious signs of disease. In the 21st century, how you feel is no longer an accurate gauge of your health.

Worldwide, the number of people who will become victims to various forms of cancer and other oxidative stress free radical diseases is growing. The threats that cause free radical disease are also growing.

As the old saying goes, "A picture is worth a thousand words." So let's try this illustration: Think about rust. Rust is oxidative stress on metal. Although the process is not identical for human cells, a similar process attacks and decays your cells. I grew up in Detroit where we often referred to our cars as having cancer. The process of rust eating away at your car is free radical oxidative stress–the same process that eats away at your cells. In "The Solution" section of this book, we will discuss some ways you can help your body cope with free radical oxidative stress.

References
1. Demmig-Adams B, Adams WW, III. Antioxidants in photosynthesis and human nutrition. *Science.* 2002;298(5601):2149-2153.
2. Di Monte DA, Lavasani M, Manning-Bog AB. Environmental factors in Parkinson's disease. *Neurotoxicology.* 2002;23(4-5):487-502.
3. Di Monte DA. The environment and Parkinson's disease: is the nigrostriatal system preferentially targeted by neurotoxins? *Lancet Neurol.* 2003;2(9):531-538.
4. Packer L, Colman C. *The Antioxidant Miracle.* John Wiley & Sons, Inc, New York, 1999.
5. American Cancer Society. *Cancer: Facts and Figures.* 2004. http://www.cancer.org/docroot/pro/content/pro_1_1_Cancer_Statistics_2004_presentation.asp

Chapter 4
The Illusion of Health: "I feel fine"

As the saying goes, "perception is everything." When I was lecturing in New Zealand in 2003, I decided to take a look at the Web sites that had information from the New Zealand government about the health of their citizens. In the first edition of my book, I gave you stats from an earlier data gathering. Below are the most recent as of the time of printing this edition.

NEW ZEALAND

Do You Think You are Well?

58% say their health is excellent or very good, but...

- 16% have asthma

- 60% are seeing their doctors 2-5 times a year

- 69% had taken at least one prescription drug during the last year

–New Zealand Health Survey, 1998[1]

Remember: As we discussed in the previous chapter, being symptom-free is not the same as being healthy.

As you can see from the numbers, 58% of New Zealanders think they are healthy. However, when you read the additional statistics, you see this simply cannot be. If 58% of New Zealanders are healthy, that means that 42% of the population is not, and that would be truly extraordinary if it were true. As you can see from doing the math yourself, many New Zealanders like people everywhere think they are healthy if they are symptom-free. You don't take drugs if you are healthy and apparently 69% of New Zealanders have in the year of the survey. Why would 60% need to see their doctors 2-5 times per year if they are healthy? Outside of an annual check, which is always prudent, "the healthy have no need for a physician." Oops! There goes that statistic!

From this data, we learn that New Zealanders who are not well think they are healthy only because they are symptom-free, even though they realize drugs control their symptoms. Unfortunately, this is the perception among most people of every country. They believe the absence of symptoms is wellness. It is also the opinion among all too many doctors. However, in the 21st century, this way of thinking is no longer correct.

Please understand I am not singling out New Zealand. This misperception of health is universal. The New Zealand government simply provided a good example from the National Survey program. I commend the New Zealand government for their efforts to recognize health issues and thereby improve the health of their citizens.

The words "I feel fine" may be some of the most dangerous words in any language when it comes to health care.

When a virus, parasite or bacteria enters your body, you feel fine. As a cancer grows in your body, you feel fine. But that does not mean you are "fine."

Most Americans you meet believe themselves to be healthy. Without major investigation, we can burst that balloon in a heartbeat. According to the American Gastroenterological Association, Americans report more than 81 million cases of chronic digestive problems each year.[2] These people feel fine and consider themselves healthy since various over-the-counter (OTC) non-prescription drugs or prescription drugs are managing their symptoms.

More commonly known is the fact that one out of every two Americans will get heart disease. Once again there is a perception problem. Everyone thinks it's the "other person" who is in the 50% that will suffer heart disease. About half of those who have their first heart attack will never have another because they will die from the first one. About half of those will have no warning or symptoms. They "feel fine" before they drop dead. More frequently, seemingly healthy individuals (including athletes) are having fatal heart attacks. Heart disease isn't just about diet or lack of exercise. It is a free radical oxidative stress disease.

There is an unrealistic perception of health shared by most people. Nearly everyone I speak with these days is concerned about aging. No one wants to grow old faster than necessary. No one wants to deal with cellular and system breakdown earlier than they have to. Again, antioxidants play a key role in preventing this process. Oxidative stress is the principal cause of premature aging.

Perhaps we can make headway by appealing to those who may think they are healthy but are concerned more about aging than they are about their overall health. The prescription is the same, and it doesn't matter how we get people to take care of themselves and protect themselves against free radical stress–as long as they do it!

> **"Scientific studies continue to indicate that we are getting too few antioxidants in our diet alone."**
>
> – Ramberg, J. *Glycoscience & Nutrition* 2001 2(16)[3]

The bar chart (Plate 2) compares the antioxidant content of a raw carrot versus one that has been cooked. This data tells us much about what we're eating. If I were to show you a chart on 1,000 different foods, each bar chart would be slightly different, but the trend would be exactly the same. If you heat-treat a food, it will lose most or even all of its nutritional value.[4]

Now look at this bar chart again: As a child, I was told that eating a carrot helped my eyes. The nutrients in a carrot that help your eyes are vitamin A and the carotenoids, such as beta-carotene. As you can see by looking at (Plate 2), vitamin A becomes nearly non-existent when the carrot is cooked. The majority of people cook their carrots. But human beings were designed to eat them raw.

In New Zealand, due to cooking habits "*al dente*," an important question was for people to know at what temperature these foods were tested. Generally, the less heat you use, the more nutrition you will retain so *al dente* is the best way. But since it is clear that any amount of heat treatment depletes nutrition from any food, let's not quibble too much about temperature. Besides, even when food is in its raw, fresh and natural state, you will still not get enough nutrition to cope with the increased stresses of our current century.

You must understand this point: We do not get enough nutrition from food in any nutritional category, but particularly in antioxidant value.

Oxidative Stress Revisited

Now let's see just how serious the oxidative stress threat is:

Since 1930, more than 75,000 synthetic chemicals have been introduced into our environment.[5] There are probably far more chemical compounds than that, because when two synthetic compounds meet in water and sunlight, they often create a new, totally unexpected compound. Thus, there really is no way to know with certainty how many potentially dangerous compounds exist on our planet today.

It's shocking to learn that only about 7% of those 75,000 synthetic chemicals have been tested for safety in adults, and only about 3% have been tested for safety in our children.[5] (Bear in mind that the environment today is completely different than the environment our bodies were designed to exist in.)

No one can avoid exposure to synthetic chemicals and toxins, regardless of where they may be. The United States Centers for Disease Control and Prevention have tested randomly chosen people around the world to see if any of them actually had toxins in their blood. This test for only 27 toxins out of a potential 75,000+ was conducted for the first time in the year 2000.[6] There were measurable, and sometimes significant, amounts of all 27 toxins evaluated, including mercury, heavy metals and the breakdown products of pesticides and plastics. (When heated, plastics produce dangerous chemicals. This process will be addressed in greater detail in "The Solution" section of this book.)

On January 30, 2003, the Environmental Working Group (EWG) published "Body Burden–The Pollution in People,"[7] the first study to thoroughly analyze the amounts of synthetic chemicals in the human body. The EWG found a disturbing average of 91 different chemical agents in the people they tested. Worse, they believe that our body burdens are on the rise.

On September 23, 2003, they published the first nationwide study on chemical fire retardants in breast milk: "Mother's Milk. Record Levels of Toxic Fire Retardants Found in American Mothers' Breast Milk."[8] This study, which included mothers from all over the United States, revealed unexpectedly high levels of brominated fire retardants in every participant tested. Furthermore, breast milk levels of these potentially neurotoxic chemicals were 75 times higher, on average, than levels reported from recent European studies.

In 2004, EWG continued their excellent work with an alert about toxic fire retardant chemicals in household dust. To ensure there is no misunderstanding on this issue, what follows is an exact quote from their study.

"In the first nationwide tests for brominated fire retardants in house dust, the EWG found unexpectedly high levels of these neurotoxic chemicals in every home sampled. The average level of brominated fire retardants measured in dust from nine homes was more than 4,600 parts per billion (ppb). A tenth sample, collected in a home where products with fire retardants were recently removed, contained more than 41,000 ppb of brominated fire retardants–twice as high as the maximum level previously reported by any dust study worldwide."

Like PCBs, their long-banned chemical relatives, the brominated fire retardants known as PBDEs (polybrominated diphenyl ethers) are persistent in the environment and bioaccumulative, building up in people's bodies over a lifetime. In minute doses they and other brominated fire retardants impair attention, learning, memory and behavior in laboratory animals.

EWGs test results indicate that consumer products, not industrial releases, are the most likely sources of the rapid buildup of PBDEs in people, animals and the environment, which has been documented by tests from Europe to the Arctic. Scientists now recognize that indoor environmental contamination, including contaminants accumulating in household dust, pose a substantial health risk to the population. Our findings raise concerns that children may ingest significant amounts of toxic fire retardants via dust, and indicate that the impending federal phase-out of two PBDEs doesn't go far enough to protect Americans.[9]

Over the next few years, the Centers for Disease Control (CDC) will eventually have tested for 100 toxins. At the current rate of testing, it would take CDC 2,778 years to test just the synthetic chemicals known at this moment. I applaud the CDC for conducting the first test, but I think they need to speed things up a bit–don't you? Their attitude has been appropriate for their mission–a sort of "not to worry, everything is under control" attitude. After all, they are the Centers for Disease Control, so how could it be otherwise?

We're All Toxic

Regardless of the CDC's posture, we can conclude that we are all toxic. One-hundred percent of toxic presence is serious regardless of the specific toxins' levels. Government doesn't know how to fix this problem. Industry, with a few sterling exceptions, doesn't want to deal with it. You can indeed take in small amounts of poison daily before you will eventually die, but that is the wrong way of thinking if you care about yourself or others.

All human beings are genetically and chemically unique. An amount of toxin that has little effect on one person may have profound effect on another. As far as I am concerned, humans were physically designed to live on a pristine, pollution-free planet. Therefore, no amount of toxin is an "acceptable level."

The reality is that we are all carrying toxins, and they will have varying effects on each of us. I would also point out two additional facts: First, we have too little data on the effects of toxins as they relate to the onset of disease to say that they are not a problem. Second, being symptom-free is no longer an accurate gauge of your health. (Sound familiar?)

In defense of CDC, I feel compelled to point out that it is their job to say, "Not to worry, everything is fine and under control"–even if it's not. What else can they say? No politician seems to have the courage to attempt to tackle the problem. Failure on any major issue can mean political suicide. No President can solve the problems with our environment in only eight years. For a politician to say they are going to fix the problems of our environment and then fail would spawn political ammunition for the opposing party to use against them in the next election. So they simply avoid any mention of these problems. Or worse, they mislead the public into thinking they care and have accomplished something substantial, when, in fact, they have not done so. It is also important to reiterate that this is a global issue, so we need politicians in every country to participate.

Any politician in any country at any level who cares enough about the people who elected him or her and has the courage to tackle this problem will have my immediate and enthusiastic support and assistance.

Even scientists who have gone to the North Pole have found pesticides and industrial chemicals in this remote region. Polar bears are showing alarming levels of toxins in their tissues that threaten their very existence.[10]

There are no farms, villages, industry or people at the North Pole. Yet toxins created in populated areas can be found in one of the most desolate places on Earth. Other scientists who went to the South Pole found farm pesticides and industrial chemicals in the fatty tissues of penguins.

Why in the fatty tissues? Most toxins are fat-soluble. The more fat you have, the more toxins you are able to store. (That alone is a reason to shed body fat!) Fish in all waterways tested thus far have been found with pesticides and industrial toxins in their bodies too. This includes fresh water and salt water, warm water and cold water, Pacific, Atlantic, Indian Ocean, river and lake water. There are no exceptions. No matter where you may be on this planet, you cannot escape toxins. I will go into detail on this in Chapter 5.

A Tragic Loss
The actor Michael Landon, a fine human being, gave millions of people pleasure with his acting and directing. I remember his last appearance on the Johnny Carson Show some years ago. He was in incredible condition and looked like an athlete. He had been eating right and exercising. He admitted that he had never looked better or felt better in his entire life and was certain he would beat the pancreatic cancer his doctors had diagnosed. However with pancreatic cancer at that time, one had a less than 1% chance of living more than 90 days. Despite Mr. Landon's efforts, regardless of how good he felt or how healthy he seemed to be, he was dead in fewer than 90 days, a tragic loss to all of us.

Maybe using this example of this fine man will help others to prevent disease. I draw on Michael Landon as an example since so many people make the same mistakes. They don't take care of their health just because they are symptom-free, or they look good, or they feel good. They think, therefore, that there are no threats to their health. As mentioned earlier, cancers do not start in a day, a week or a month. It is a progressive process that goes on for years before your body finally cannot cope with it any longer.

Let's look at another example: When bacteria or virus invades your body, you feel fine. In fact, you may feel fine for days before your body begins to combat (perhaps not very effectively) the microbes that have entered your body. By the time you know a virus or bacteria has invaded, it's too late. That's one key reason it's so important to keep your immune system at peak function at all times. You cannot do this through diet alone, and you cannot wait until you have been diagnosed with a health problem.

You must be proactive about your body and your health. You must always think as though you are under attack, because in fact you are. Think defensively. Eat defensively. Take care of yourself properly, and you will maximize your potential for a long and healthy life.

References
1. Abernathy P. New Zealand Health Survey (October 1996 to September 1997). New Zealand Ministry of Healthy, 20 July 1998: http://www.stats.govt.nz/domino/

external/pasfull/pasfull.nsf/0/4c2567ef00247c6a4c2568490008a1fb?Open Document

2. The American Gastroenterological Association. Consumer Survey Results – Know your Gut. March 16, 2003: http://www.gastro.org/corescore/consumerSurvey.html
3. Ramberg J, Vennum EP, Boyd S, et al. Vitamins and minerals: consolidated review of the potential benefits. *GlycoScience & Nutrition.* 2001;2(16):1-17.
4. Ramberg J, McAnalley BH. From the farm to the kitchen table: a review of the nutrient losses in foods. *GlycoScience & Nutrition.* 2002;3(5):1-12.
5. Moyers B, Jones S. Trade Secrets: A Moyers Report. Public Affairs Television Inc., 2001: http://www.pbs.org/tradesecrets/
6. Centers for Disease Control and Prevention. *Second National Report on Human Exposure to Environmental Chemicals.* Department of Health and Human Services: 2003. http://www.cdc.gov/nceh/dls/report/PDF/NatExpRep.pdf
7. Houlihan J, Wiles R, Thayer K, and Gray S. *Body burden. The pollution in people.* Environmental Working Group: 1-30-2003. http://www.ewg.org/reports/body burden/
8. Lunder S and Sharp R. *Mothers' milk. Record levels of toxic fire retardants found in American mothers' breast milk.* Environmental Working Group: Washington, D.C., 2003. http://www.ewg.org/reports/mothersmilk/
9. Sharp R and Lunder S. *In the Dust. Toxic Fire Retardants in American Homes.* Environmental Working Group: Washington, D.C., 2004: http://www.ewg.org/reports/inthedust/
10. Guynup S. *Arctic Life Threatened by Toxic Chemicals, Groups Say.* National Geographic Today, October 8, 2002.

Chapter 5
Toxins in Your Water

I have been warning people in my lectures about toxins in their water for more than 17 years. For example, for all these years I have been recommending that you limit your intake of seafood to only once per month. Most people hearing that don't like my recommendation–most of them are consumers who love seafood (as I do) or people involved in some way with the seafood industry, from fisheries to grocery stores and restaurants. Since people didn't like hearing what I said about toxins in our water, they were certain I had to be wrong. And, of course, they assumed that the data that I had compiled 17 years ago was "insufficient–simply a theory and personal recommendation."

Since then the data has mounted, and in 2003 it was widely publicized that certain fish must be eaten sparingly. In fact, as you will read in this chapter, the recommendation from various experts was once per month for salmon and other fish that have higher body fat, which is bad, and therefore also a higher content of essential fatty acids (EFAs), which is very healthful. EFAs, also referred to as the omega fatty acids, are essential to human life, and the fatter the fish (like salmon), the more EFAs it contains. But the toxins that cause disease, birth defects, reduced brain function, development disorders, neuromuscular disease, cancers, loss of fertility and feminizing effects in males are all fat-soluble, so the more fat, the more toxin, and more.

In March 2004, the U.S. Food and Drug Administration (FDA) reiterated this warning to limit the consumption of certain fish. FDA issued the advisory about mercury and pregnancy, saying pregnant women should avoid consuming certain fish. Those fish included the larger fish such as shark, swordfish, king mackerel and tilefish because they might contain levels of mercury that could lead to brain damage in a developing fetus.[1] Mercury is a serious problem, one most people know about, but in this book I'll name others the FDA and the media haven't told you about.

Industry leaders say environmentalists are overreacting and are quick to stereotype anyone with an environmental concern. I have no desire to harm any industry or put any jobs at risk, which is the principal criticism by industry against environmentalism. Industries that do not want to take responsibility for the suffering and death caused by their actions are generally quick in their attempts to discredit environmentalists by saying we are reactionaries or anarchists or worse.

The word environmentalist, thanks to vilification by industry leaders and their spokesmen, now conjures up a popular image of a wild-eyed, sandal-wearing anarchist who has never washed his uncombed hair and beard and advocates an end to capitalism.

Stereotyping is wrong because it is so often inaccurate. Unfortunately, however, it is also a reality of life. So let me address this stereotype right now:

I have never had long hair or a beard, even in the 1960s when all my peers had them. Regarding sandals, I have only worn them to the beach. I am not an anarchist, nor do I desire our civilization to come to an end with all of us reverting to Stone Age technologies. I love some of the wonders and conveniences of the modern world, but we must learn to integrate them with nature and eliminate the products of science that are harmful while retaining and creating technologies that will benefit life on this beautiful blue planet without destructive or harmful side effects.

I would be absolutely delighted–in fact, thrilled beyond words!–to work with any industry or politician to help them understand how to create jobs and increase profits by making changes that can clean up our ailing planet and help prevent disease. We can only solve our problems and protect future generations if we stop bickering with each other and work cooperatively toward common goals. There are industries that must be established in response to the current and future needs of all the people of this world. Captains of industry are simply missing a trillion-dollar opportunity!

How I wish I could counsel them, to advise them how to be profitable and actually increase the health of all living creatures on this planet. Industry leaders, as well as government officials, would be surprised to learn how much we can do to improve the condition of our world. I offer many suggestions for you and for them in Chapters 11, 12 and 13. This book is not intended to provide every detail of every problem and its solutions, but any government official or industry leader who is willing to try to make a difference will command my undivided attention and full cooperation.

If I had the funds, I would start several new industries myself to help our world. They would employ more people and help increase our total Gross National Product (GNP). But I am only one man, and I cannot do this alone. However, these ideas are not unrealistic–they represent a very real business opportunity.

Now, on to the topics in this chapter. Each of those listed below merits their own university textbooks. The purpose of this book is to alert you and educate you just enough so that you will understand why you need to take action, and then what actions you can personally take. Thus, I must unfortunately be brief, and I cannot possibly list every toxin and their effects in every way currently known. I hope, however, that this chapter will be sufficient to put you on the right track.

What we'll examine in this chapter:
- Toxins in seafood
- The effects of toxins on aquatic life
- Toxic waste produced by industry
- Toxic waste produced by government
- Untreated sewage from cities and countries
- Feminizing chemicals in the world's water supply
- Reductions in male fertility worldwide

Connect the Drops (of Water)
Most people are totally unaware of what is actually in the water worldwide. Although an occasional news story shows a factory dumping something disgusting and nasty into the water, most people don't think about the water all over the planet being affected by this incident.

All water on Earth is connected, either by direct currents in the waterway, by underground water flow or by precipitation and weather fronts. (Plate 3).[2]

There is no possibility of water anywhere on the planet that will not be affected in some way. Although some countries have made a little progress in helping to control industrial waste and pesticide usage, it really is no more than a drop in the ocean. (Yes, the pun is intentional!)

Governments worldwide must take action to solve our environmental problems. All elected and appointed officials must realize the seriousness of the threats to life on planet Earth and begin to work diligently together to solve these problems. Thus far, environmentalists have been unsuccessful in alerting officials or the media (and therefore the public) to the enormity and seriousness of the issues that threaten the very future of life in our world. Let's be clear:

At this time, most government leaders do not work toward solving these crucial environmental issues.

In context of these issues, we can group political leaders into four broad categories:
1. **Those who care and know the issues but cannot get enough support to implment the changes necessary.**
2. **Those who are totally ignorant of the issues, but would work honestly and conscientiously if they were aware of this information.**
3. **Those who know some or perhaps all of the issues but don't care, focusing all of their efforts on getting re-elected no matter the costs.**
4. **Those who know some or perhaps all of the issues but profit from the industries that cause pollution by accepting favors from them or by getting votes from workers employed by industries that harm our planet. If it doesn't affect them personally and immediately, they simply do not care.**

We need to work with leaders from the first and second groups and compel those in groups three and four to take their obligations to us and our planet seriously. Once the public understands the true extent of the threats, we can only hope that they may change their voting habits.

The news stories we hear are typically press releases that government officials and industry leaders want us to have. They want us to believe that they've made a particular step or strides toward cleaning up the environment–particularly prior to elections. However, the fact is that the overwhelming majority of waste and toxic material created in the world today is still being dumped directly into our environment. Yes, there are good politicians who do care and actually try to correct these problems, but they are unfortunately a minority of elected and appointed officials.

I also believe that there are good men and women in governments who simply do not know how serious the threats to life on this planet are and therefore do nothing because they are not aware of the problem or its extent. Those officials need this book. In addition, there are leaders in many nations who have no regard for human life and give no thought to the future of our world. There are also politicians that are selfish and short-sighted, caring only about their terms of office or their political parties. They don't care how their actions may affect the rest of the world.

Some governments struggle to keep their populations employed, and because of that struggle, they allow industries to cut corners just to create and/or save jobs. And some countries are so poor and desperate that simply keeping their populations alive takes 100% of their efforts and financial resources, so the environment receives absolutely no attention at all. I believe there may be leaders of these destitute nations who, if they had the information and the resources, would work to clean up the environment in their geographical areas.

Very poor nations typically have uncontrolled population growth and inadequate food supplies. To feed their people, government leaders in these nations believe they must use chemicals like pesticides over the short term. They still use chemicals like DDT even though this pesticide has been declared illegal in more prosperous nations.

It is not my intent to vilify any particular nation, but since I cannot discuss every country and what is wrong in each individually, I will simply offer a few examples to help you understand the nature of the problems we must face.

Mercury Rising

Brazil is one of those struggling nations that can barely make ends meet for most of its population. In Brazil, the government allows gold miners to use a particular method of mining along the Amazon River that results in tons of mercury entering the environment every year. To illustrate how every action has consequences beyond its localized effects, this mercury runs into the Amazon River, which then runs into the Atlantic Ocean and eventually reaches all of our water systems.

As you study the water current (Plate 3)[2], notice how mercury contamination from the Amazon affects the Atlantic Ocean. While that effect is short-term, it affects the world over the long term since all water is connected in some way. The irresponsible release of mercury is one of the biggest single sources of mercury contamination in the world's seafood and water supply. The miners who actually do the mining that produces the mercury get the equivalent of about one-hundred U.S. dollars a month in exchange for poisoning the Earth, allowing them to barely keep their families fed. But what is the cost to life on our planet? Can't we find a different way for these miners to earn $100 (or more) per month–a way that won't harm our planet?

In 1992, a world summit on the environment took place–ironically in Brazil. The United States did not join that group. However Brazil agreed "to clean up its act." So why is this harmful practice continuing? Why is Brazil still destroying thousands of acres of Amazon rain forests every single day? Trees are the lungs of our planet, and without them most life would cease to exist. The soil that becomes available after destroying trees is good during only one farming season, and then it becomes wasteland. Can't we help Brazil and all the other Brazils of the world feed their populations more intelligently? "Give a man a fish, and you feed him for a day; teach a man to fish, and you feed him for a lifetime."

Were you already aware of this issue? We must not wait until our grandchildren are gasping for air before we confront this problem and similar ones head-on.

Being an objectivist, I feel compelled to find and report some positive news about Brazil as well. Raytheon Corporation, makers of the Patriot missile, has been awarded a $1.4 billion contract from the Brazilian government to build and operate a radar-based environmental monitoring system for the Amazon River basin. This system could give us crucially important data about the Amazon rain forest that could lead to major strides in preserving life throughout the world. In this case, we will have to wait and see what eventually happens. (You can read more about this system on Raytheon's Web site).

Both human and industrial wastes are dumped into waterways worldwide every day. Most countries just cannot afford to take the proper steps. Some are governed by people who simply do not know or understand the issues. Some are simply too corrupt. For example, the former Soviet Union dumped raw nuclear waste from their nuclear submarines into its harbor at Vladivostok, putting radioactive waste into the Sea of Japan–"hot" waste that eventually found its way into the Pacific Ocean. Are the Russians still doing this dumping now even though the old Soviet Union has been dissolved?

Acknowledging the current regime's economic problems and how much the cost to clean up this situation would be, it would be logical to assume they still are. But in their defense, I must say I have not seen it, nor do I have irrefutable data to prove that they have stopped the practice either.

Russia desperately struggles to survive as a nation. Their economy simply has no funds available for the environment. Other nations in Europe (some with sufficient funds) have placed no restrictions on the amount of pesticide that flows into their waterways. We desperately need to stop making war on each other for the same old, petty reasons and start making war on the toxins in our environment. Everyone everywhere must work together, or we may indeed lose the war to save our planet.

And before we move on, let's remember that this is a global problem. Recent studies show that rivers in Europe–for example the legendary, naturally beautiful Rhine–have now become a dumping ground for pesticide runoff.[3]

DDT–Gone? Not Hardly!

Once again, I cannot detail every pesticide and their uses or effects in this book, so I will start with one that is familiar to everyone. Around the world, there are nations that currently have absolutely no restriction on the use of DDT. Some of these nations' produce, such as grapes that we consume off-season, plus other products made from that same produce–like the majority of the world's wines, which are made from grapes–are drenched in DDT. (Have you ever considered what your favorite wine goes through before it reaches your lips?)

DDT was made illegal for use by the U.S. and other progressive nations in 1972, but the number-one producer of DDT in the world remains the United States. DDT is still sold to nations around the world where there are no restrictions on its use. The American public has been intentionally or unintentionally (I have no way of confirming it either way) led to believe that the politicians who pushed to have DDT made illegal for use in the U.S. were ridding the world of it, and therefore correcting at least the immediate threat that environmentalists were up in arms about. Unfortunately, DDT is still pervasive throughout the world environment, including North America.

Between 1930 (when first used) and its ban in 1972, approximately 675,000 tons of DDT were applied in the U.S. alone. Chemicals like DDT do not break down easily. In a study conducted during 1992 and 1993, DDT was found in 25% of homes twenty years after it had been prohibited from use. Toxic agents designed to degrade quickly outdoors in the presence of sunlight, moisture and bacteria can survive for years when tracked indoors on shoes and trapped deep in the pile of carpets.[4] The half-life of DDT in humans is eight years. That means it would take much more than 16 years for DDT taken into your body today to be eliminated. Sixteen years would actually be the minimal time period required for DDT to affect you, but, since we are still constantly exposed to DDT, we cannot calculate its long-term effects.

DDT and many other chemicals in the environment make a strong case for the attention of the United Nations. Whatever your political beliefs and despite the U.S. government's reluctance to deal unilaterally with world environmental issues, America must lead the UN to help those nations too poor to control pollution. The United States must also take action against those countries that are too corrupt to spend the money to help eradicate these problems. Environmental toxins are truly weapons of mass destruction, but rather than taking life in the blink of an eye, they take years to cause the pain and suffering that lead to death.

Proponents of DDT's manufacture and use say it has saved more lives than any other chemical since it kills mosquitoes that carry malaria, plus other dangerous parasites. The people who profit from its sale and those who support them will say and do anything to discredit those who want DDT totally banned from our world. There are always at least two sides to any story, however. This debate brings up a very complex moral issue– especially for me.

It's a fact that pesticides like DDT will effectively kill mosquitoes (and other parasites) that can cause disease. This large-scale extermination effort can save many lives in populations of individuals who may later die from disease due to poor nutrition and often-nonexistent sanitation. There are those who say we need to let those populations naturally thin out because their cultures will not take action to responsibly control their own population growth. They reason: Let nature take care of the population problem for us.

I cannot take issue with either camp since both use valid reasoning. But I believe human life should always be the first choice. This belief sets up a conflict within me, because chemicals like DDT are extremely harmful to life on this planet over the long term, while being extremely helpful to life in the near term.

It isn't just the definite extinction by DDT of birds of prey–the primary reason for the outlawing of DDT in North America–but the long-term feminizing effect of a metabolite of DDT called DDE, which I believe over time will put the human population at risk of extinction. It is the age-old question, "Do the needs of the many outweigh the needs of the few?"

From my perspective, we are either part of the solution, or we are part of the problem. We cannot be both. If objective third-party data indicates a threat to human and animal life, there is clearly a problem. However my, opinion is just that–an opinion. You are certainly entitled to draw your own conclusions.

Live with Other Life Forms

I believe we can use non-toxic methods to control parasites. Safe pesticides can be made from plant materials that would not be intended for human consumption, so the soil needed to grow it wouldn't have to be the best topsoil. This suggestion won't sit well with those who profit from DDT, but if we could convince them to switch to safer insecticides, they could eventually profit financially while the whole planet profited from the resultant life-saving change. There are new and environmentally aware specialists in pest control–not pest eradication–that have new, safer methods than chemicals like DDT. I believe in the next few years we will see industries evolve around these safer and more natural methods. I am not a fan of mosquitoes or other parasites. But insects play a crucial role in the world ecosystem, so we can't just wipe out whatever offends us. We must learn to live with nature.

Let's examine this issue more closely. I will offer more facts to help you to decide where you stand on this issue.

Experts disagree about whether DDT causes cancer in humans. I believe it does, but once again, that is only my opinion. Of course, both sides believe they are right. We know DDT causes cancer in animals. Increased tumor production in the liver and lungs has been observed in test animals. Former U.S. Assistant Surgeon General Dr. David Rall says, "Every chemical known to cause cancer in experimental animals also causes cancer in humans. While some species are more sensitive to toxic effects than others, laboratory studies have proven to be good predictors of health effects in humans."[5]

Dr. Rall, now at the National Institute for Occupational Safety and Health (NIOSH), presented additional evidence for admissibility of animal carcinogenesis when he addressed the causes of human cancer in his peer-reviewed publication, which also supports the scientific policy of the International Agency for Research on Cancer. The prevailing opinion in carcinogenesis is that agents shown to be carcinogenic in animals that do not have safety studies in humans also present a cancer risk to humans. Rall stated, "Experimental evidence indicates that there are more physiological, biochemical and metabolic similarities between laboratory animals and humans than there are differences. These similarities increase the probability that results observed in a laboratory setting will predict similar results for humans." Clearly, the accumulated experience in the field for carcinogenesis supports this concept.[6] (I will quote David Rall again in chapter 6 because this important point merits additional emphasis.)

Data from the International Agency for Research on Cancer (IARC) Monograph Series[7] and the National Toxicology Program Report, as well as the Department of Health and Human Services' reports on carcinogenesis,[8] show a long list of chemicals at first shown to be cancer-causing only in animals, but that were subsequently shown to cause cancer in humans too. If you are interested, this information is in the public domain and is strong enough to make any reasonable person understand that if a substance is toxic to lab animals, it is also very likely toxic to people. There simply isn't enough time, interest or money to test more than 75,000 synthetic compounds to see if each of them causes cancer in human beings.

In addition, there have been several human studies to consider how DDT relates specifically to cancer. In one study, a significant association between long-term, high DDT exposure and pancreatic cancers in chemical workers was suggested. (In the interest of objectivity, there were questions raised about the reliability of the medical records of a large proportion of the cancer cases studied. Once again both sides believe they are correct. This is another case where more scientific investigation is needed.)[9,10]

We know DDT can affect people and other animals in various ways. DDT is a neurotoxin (nerve poison) for insects, and the chemical is also known to affect the human nervous system adversely. (I will refer frequently in this book to the effects of toxins as they relate to body mass.) Obviously adult humans can withstand far more toxin than insects and still survive. However, since nervous system disorders are on the rise, we have to learn if there is any connection with DDT or similar chemicals. Again, more study is needed, so let's look at what we already know for sure:

Exposure to DDT and its by-product metabolites, DDE and DDD, occurs mostly from eating foods containing small amounts of these compounds–particularly meat, fish and poultry. High levels of DDT can affect the nervous system, causing excitability, tremors and seizures.[9] High levels can also adversely affect the liver and kidneys.[9] In women, DDE can reduce the duration of lactation and result in an increased chance of having a baby prematurely. More than 30 years after its U.S. ban, DDT, DDE, and DDD have been found in at least 441 of the 1,613 National Priorities List sites identified by the Environmental Protection Agency (EPA). DDT and its metabolites are apparently not breaking down as its manufacturers either intended or represented.

Another area of both concern and controversy is DDT's potential to damage human chromosomes. DDT showed positive results in only one out of 11 mutagenicity assays in various cell cultures and organisms.[9] Results of *in vitro* and *in vivo* genotoxicity assays for chromosomal aberrations, however, indicated that DDT was genotoxic in 8 out of 12 cases, and weakly genotoxic in one case.[9]

DDT also seems to lower the cognitive (thinking) ability of lab animals. However, based on data currently available, once again the levels of exposure the average adult would get are not sufficient to cause that same effect in humans. In my view, more study is required.

DDT and DDE are both classified as xeno-estrogens. These are chemicals that mimic the hormone estrogen in animals and humans. This is a highly controversial area of study. Xeno-estrogens cause a feminizing affect in animals and are suspected to do the same in humans. Almost no one wants to discuss this issue, but, since this book is "telling it like it really is," we will discuss this sensitive topic later in this chapter.

All pesticides–not just DDT–end up in the water table. That means they end up in anything that lives in or drinks from the water. In short, we're including all life on planet Earth. DDT is very highly toxic to many aquatic invertebrate species.[11,12] Early developmental stages are more susceptible than adults to DDT.[11] The reversibility of some effects, as well as the development of some resistance, may be possible in some aquatic invertebrates.[12] Remember too that most toxins in humans have more serious effects during growth stages that in adulthood.

DDT is very highly toxic to fish species as well. Many fish have been tested, including Coho salmon, rainbow trout, northern pike, black bullhead, bluegill sunfish, largemouth bass, walleye, fathead minnow and channel catfish.[12] In separate studies, other fish have been tested and also showed higher levels of DDT than needed to affect the hatching of eggs. These included largemouth bass and guppies.[11] It is reported that DDT levels of one nanogram (one billionth of a gram) per liter–that's far less than in all the fish mentioned above–in Lake Michigan were sufficient to affect the hatching of Coho salmon eggs.[13]

DDT may be moderately toxic to some amphibian species, and larval stages are probably more susceptible than adults.[11,14] In addition to acute toxic effects, DDT may bioaccumulate significantly in fish and other aquatic species, leading to long-term exposure. This exposure occurs mainly through uptake from sediment and water into aquatic flora and fauna, as well as fish.[11] Fish uptake of DDT from the water is size-dependent, with smaller fish taking up relatively more than larger fish. This factor is due to the half-life of the chemical–a concept I'll explain later.[11]

The reported bioconcentration factor for DDT is 1,000 to 1,000,000 in various aquatic species,[15] and bioaccumulation may occur in some species at very low environmental concentrations.[12] Bioaccumulation may also result in exposure to species that prey on fish or other aquatic organisms (e.g. birds of prey).

If there is good news regarding seafood and DDT, it is that cooking, especially at high heat, can reduce (not eliminate) DDT levels in fish. This reduction occurs because the toxins are stored in fat. As you cook away the fat, you separate some of the toxins. So you should broil, bake or grill (not fry) fish after you have removed the skin and carefully trimmed the fish. Please note that doing this reduces chemicals, but not metals like mercury. So you still need to limit your intake.[16]

The manufacturers of DDT in the U.S. might defend themselves by saying that if they don't produce it, someone else will. That may be true, but the proverbial buck

has to stop somewhere. **In my opinion, there's no excuse for producing DDT. Until all governments agree to prohibit the manufacture of known toxins, the problem will simply keep getting worse.**[17]

Your senses can deceive you. Alaska is one of the most beautiful places I have ever seen. Yet, did you know that there are hundreds of toxic waste dumps in the state of Alaska? These include U.S. Super Fund sites, radioactive waste sites, sites declared contaminated by the Astrophysics Data Centers Executive Council (ADEC), chemical weapons dumps and more. Most Alaskans are totally unaware of this presence of toxic waste sites throughout their beautiful state. Fishermen who catch fish and crab from the cold waters off the coast of Alaska generally do not know about the toxins that have been buried along the coastline, as well as inland, in Alaska. *Human senses were designed to detect things that occur naturally on our planet, and we just cannot detect the great majority of synthetic threats.*

Contaminated seafood, pregnancy and early development

A study was done on pregnant women who had consumed fish. It seems that their children have the highest rate thus far studied of developmental disorders.[18] Consumption of Great Lakes fish is a common factor among these women. Sadly, this connection between developmental problems in children–including impaired or slow learning–is not isolated to the Great lakes.[16] Other studies indicate a strong correlation between learning problems, ADD and ADHD and the intake of chemicals found in our water.[19,20,21,22,23] Another interesting study on behavioral problems in children as it related to toxins in fish was called the Grandmother Rat Study. We do not know why, but negative behavior continued among rat pups into the third generation, even though the second-generation mothers had not been exposed to PCBs.[23]

How can this be? Scientists aren't sure, but the suggestion is that this problem is far more serious than we had thought. Can you begin to see why I am so concerned for our future generations?

Fish have no choice but to immerse their bodies in water, and whatever is in that water goes straight into them. They are designed to get their oxygen by passing water through their tissues 24 hours a day. They cannot help but be saturated with whatever may be in the water. Remember, too, that big fish eat little fish, so the bigger the fish (such as a shark), typically the greater the concentration of toxins that will be present. The concentration level can vary with certain toxins in specific fish. However, when it comes to toxic metals like mercury, for example, bigger fish tend to be more toxic overall. Some toxins like DDT are actually concentrated more highly in smaller and younger fish due to the half-life of the chemicals.

What about fertility?

Scientists in Denmark completed a 20-year study on fertility in males and found that human males are becoming less fertile, with lower sperm motility and lower sperm counts.[24] These results correlate directly with the quantity of feminizing chemicals known as xeno-estrogens in our waterways and, consequently, also in the fish and marine mammals.

Aquatic life includes marine mammals as well as the birds that feed on that aquatic life. As mentioned earlier, this was the reason DDT was made illegal in the U.S. Birds of prey like the American bald eagle were being driven to extinction by 1970 due to the toxic effects of this pesticide. In addition, DDT and DDE cause severe eggshell thinning in birds. Those most severely affected are once again the birds of prey since they are at the top of the food chain. That is an important concept to bear in mind, since we humans, too, are at the top of our own food chain.

By continually consuming fish and small mammals with low levels of DDT that is not excreted or degraded, the toxin accumulates and becomes concentrated in the tissues of these animals. The offspring of contaminated birds have a very high mortality rate due to incomplete gestation within the thin eggshells. Rachel Carson, author of the monumental book, **Silent Spring,** made a strong impression on me as a young man in the sixties with her book. She was right to sound the alarm but unfortunately incorrect when she said DDT was killing off "song birds." As I have mentioned, only birds of prey have been specifically documented, due to the feeding habits listed above. Birds of prey are part of a group called raptors, which includes the more than 250 species of hawks as well as ospreys, kites, vultures and eagles. However, there is ample documented data to tell me that DDT is doing more harm over the long term than it does good.

Mass die-offs of animals have occurred worldwide since the 1970s. Scientists have checked these die-offs to learn why dozens–and, in a few cases, hundreds–of mammals and thousands of dead and dying fish have washed up on our beaches. The scientists found that in the case of marine mammals, pesticides and industrial toxins had compromised their immune systems, and they died under normal conditions from relatively minor infections. Their bodies should have resisted infection without any problem. But their tissues were heavily laden with chemical toxins (plus metals), some of which are known to suppress immune function.

Between 1987 and 1991, dolphin and seal die-offs were recorded in the North Sea, Baltic Sea, off the eastern coast of the United States, in the Gulf of Mexico and in the Mediterranean. The carcasses of these animals were found to contain elevated levels of polychlorinated biphenyls (PCBs), dioxins and other organochlorines known to accumulate in the blubber (or lipid tissues) of large species and predators at the top of the food chain. These die-offs and an epidemic of tumors observed in green sea turtles have been linked to the cumulative buildup of PCBs and other chemicals that are believed to weaken immune systems, causing susceptibility to viral infections.[25]

Birds that live on seafood are sending us a warning. Yes, their bodies are smaller than ours, so they can tolerate fewer toxins than we can before they become diseased or go extinct. And their diet is concentrated in toxins that are accumulated in seafood. But what's happening to them should serve as an important alert for all of us, nonetheless.

Another example is the recent documentation of mass die-offs of African flamingos.

The African flamingo population is declining at the rate of about 20 percent every two decades. At this rate, the entire species will become extinct within 100 years, according to Ramesh Thampy, Director of the World Wildlife Fund's Eastern Africa Regional Program in Nakuru.[26]

The first documented mass die-off of African flamingos occurred in 1993, with an estimated 40,000 birds perishing from August to November. Two years later, about 20,000 more died. More mass deaths came in 1997, with smaller losses since. Apparently no other lake mammals or birds have been affected this severely. Pollution was a suspected cause, so researchers tested the dead birds for toxic substances. Analysis showed detectable levels of many metals known to be by-products of industry–and the area of

Africa affected has become heavily industrialized since about 1975.[26]

Tests revealed the tissue of these stilt-legged birds was burdened with zinc, copper, lead, mercury, cadmium, selenium, chromium, iron and arsenic.[26] Lead, mercury, cadmium and arsenic are just toxic, plain and simple. Zinc, copper, selenium, chromium and iron are healthful and required for life, but after reaching a certain level, they also can become toxic. According to Gideon Motelin, a veterinary pathologist at Egerton University in Nakuru, the presence of heavy metals in the bird tissues was found at levels that "threaten the very existence of the flamingos."[26]

In the interest of objectivity, I must also report other factors that must be taken into consideration. A team of German and Scottish researchers identified one additional potential killer–a potent neurotoxin produced by a type of blue-green algae. (Not the kind of blue-green algae sold as a nutritional supplement).

These scientists said they assumed that this neurotoxin, referred to as anatoxin-a, is also contributing to the die-offs since they found it in high concentrations. However, they also pointed out that the bird's detoxification capacity might be exhausted by overexposure to pesticides and heavy metals, allowing less toxic outbreaks to become lethal.[26] This die-off follows the same pattern as marine mammals, whose immune systems have been so stressed by toxins that they can no longer fight off even minor infections.

One more factor that should be food for thought: Flamingos can live for 50 years, allowing a steady, potentially deadly accumulation of toxins As I point out frequently in this book, most toxins take years before they will adversely affect us in ways our doctors can diagnose. Also keep in mind that, just like various birds of prey, the flamingo is at the top of its particular food chain. Do you sense a recurring theme here?

Aren't <u>organic, farm-raised</u> fish safe to eat?

This is a very important question. Consumers should definitely seek food sources that provide the most natural possible foods. I will reinforce this idea more than once in this book. The quick, simple definition of organic is something that is or was at one time alive. Therefore all natural food is organic, regardless of whether it comes from plant or animal and regardless of how it was grown or raised.

In a more scientific sense, organic means it contains carbon molecules. All life on planet Earth is carbon-based. My boots fit all the scientific parameters to be called organic. They are made from leather and wood, living materials composed of carbon and other molecules. They are not, however, safe, non-toxic or nutritious. Therefore, I would not recommend my boots as a food supplement.

Have I made my point that the word organic can be and has been often misused? Over the years, the general public has been led to believe that organic means cleaner, safer or even more nutritious. According to a federal survey, since fewer than 4% of Americans have a background in science, it is not surprising they would think this way.

I want to be clear in saying that almost all suppliers of foods sold as organic are reputable, honest, well-intentioned individuals who simply don't know they have been misusing the word. However, the word organic has been so misused for so long that I fully expect the definition to eventually be officially changed to fit the public perception, regardless of scientific accuracy. We will most likely see it in the dictionary that way in the near future.

When a food seller says organic, they mean that no toxins were *intentionally* used in the raising of the animals or produce. There are varying degrees in this area too. An article in *Time* magazine in 2003 stated that organic, farm-raised salmon were actually more toxic than those in the ocean. This was quite a jolt for salmon lovers and the salmon farm industry,[27] which has worked diligently and at considerable expense to provide the cleanest, most natural source of salmon possible.

Salmon has huge nutritional value. The content of essential fatty acids, protein and minerals in salmon is exceptional. However, ocean salmon are not healthy any more since they are among the fattier fish, and the toxins that cause cancer and other health issues are fat-soluble. More fat means more toxins. It is that simple. Keep this fact in mind as you select fish for your family meal.

Salmon farms had taken every precaution but did not consider the effects of what they fed the salmon. The protein meal they fed the "organic" salmon was made from a concentrate that came from ocean fish. Without realizing it, salmon farmers were concentrating the toxic content of the salmon. They were feeding their otherwise pristine fish levels of toxins far greater than they would have eaten even if they had been swimming freely in the ocean.

What can the well-intentioned salmon farmers say now? Some of them say *Time* was wrong, and that the problem isn't serious. Everything is just fine. What else can they say?

It would be a terrible shame for everyone, not just the fish farms, if they had to go out of business. What the farmers should do is simply admit that they were unaware of the problem, change the food source and continue to offer one of the best nutritional values a person can consume. Regretfully, some of the farms have not done that and remain in a state of anger and denial. Hopefully in the future, this situation will be resolved, and we will have a clean source of this excellent food, just as the organic farmers have always intended.

I would advise consumers to be cautious and skeptical when it comes to buying and eating "organic." Many types of fish are raised on organic farms, and other foods– from shrimp to beef–are raised on similar farms. Are the farms and foods produced there clean and safe? What do the food animals eat? Chances are they are exactly what they represent, but be careful: Ask questions before you buy.

What about birth defects?

Deformed fish have been reported everywhere. News commentators snicker or laugh that "Oh well, a three-eyed fish was found in Boston Harbor today." However, this isn't a laughing matter. It's a serious problem happening worldwide. And it is a very clear call to action because time is running out.

There is a definite reason that animals and fish are born deformed. We know that certain chemicals can cause birth defects in any living creature. (Yes, I said any living creature, and that includes humans). But it doesn't have to be that way.

You can easily ignore the problem if your children are born physiologically normal. But the unimaginable heartbreak of parents who are not so fortunate cannot be ignored and could be prevented in most cases by taking the proper steps. And what of the child who must suffer through life with deformities, abnormalities and deficiencies? Shouldn't we all just do our bit and change this situation for those yet unborn? Why can't everyone see how urgent the need is?

For several years, we have been hearing stories about frogs and other amphibians that have been born with multiple legs, no legs and all manner of other grotesque deformities. At first, government officials told us these abnormalities had to do with radiation from the sun, not pollution. When the public wouldn't accept that absurd story, we were subsequently told that it had to do with parasites in the water—again, not pollution. Are there parasites that can cause deformities and birth defects in frogs? Yes, but are they the cause in every case? No, I think not.

Is it mere coincidence that frogs living in areas that have been sprayed with mutagens are born mutated? What about other species with awful mutations that live in the same areas and will drink the same water or eat the animals that live in that water? Are they also the victims of frog parasites?

Let's get real: A common factor among all of these deformed and/or mutated amphibians and other species that live in the same general area and drink the same water is the level of chemical toxins found in their tissues, as well as the water. While we could provide umbrellas and sunscreen for all the frogs, or put anti-parasite medication in the water they live in, I guarantee that doing so will not prevent the mutations in these amphibians.

Remember those marine mammals that died from routine minor infections because their immune systems had been compromised by chemical toxins? Is it possible a similar reaction is occurring among the mutated frogs?

Roads to Extinction

The possibility that frogs and other species may become extinct from human-created toxins is very real. Every living creature is on this planet for a reason. Each plays a role in the total world ecosystem. Frogs help control pests like mosquitoes, and without frogs many insects would grow out of control. We must work to ensure that species do not go extinct. The human race must begin to think global, and understand that all creatures—even ones we fear or dislike—must be allowed to play their roles in the ecosystem.

Scientists have also studied birds and other animals that depend primarily on water as their food source, as well as the water source itself. We see increasing numbers of aquatic birds that are born deformed. A common birth defect among some birds now is a beak so twisted they can't feed themselves. Without humans to care for them and feed them by hand daily, they will simply die of starvation. Will we let some species become extinct because of chemicals made by humans—chemicals that we never really needed and that should not have been on this planet to begin with?

Scientists have learned that many birds now have a greatly reduced birth rate than they formerly had. Birds, alligators, turtles and other animals that live in water, as opposed to just taking an occasional drink, are having the most pronounced reduction in birth rates, especially of male offspring. One doesn't have to be a scientist to realize that without males, a species will become extinct.

But lack of male offspring is not the only problem in this general area. A new phenomenon has been observed by scientists, one few people have even yet heard about—the creation of a third, but temporary, sex known as intersex. Intersex is present when offspring are born with both male and female genitalia but are unable to reproduce.

Chemical gender confusion is further illustrated in birds. In numerous instances, female seagulls have been observed behaving like males, attempting to copulate with female gulls as they would if they were truly male. These female gulls will not allow males to approach them and are relentless (like males) in pursuing females. This is not isolated either and is commonly observed never landfills where chemicals known to be xeno-estrogens are concentrated. My theory is that these lesbian gulls were genetically conceived to be males but the influence of xeno-estrogens during gestation caused them to be born with female genitalia but male brains, if you will.

Chemicals affect our world in tragic ways we would never have imagined even a decade ago. Environmental scientists are justifiably concerned that some species may become extinct soon as a result of this phenomenon.[28]

The more body mass a living creature has, the more toxin it can tolerate before the toxin will produce a negative effect. Small creatures like seagulls, turtles and frogs will be affected more rapidly, so we will observe their changes sooner. Since they have shorter lifespans than humans, it is also easier for us to observe the birth defects and the cumulative effects of generational mutation. But the same chemicals affect us, as well.

One scientist, studying feminizing synthetic chemicals in the environment, was asked how much of a specific chemical would be needed to affect a human being. He said that the amount of estrogen–in this case, referring to synthetic chemical estrogens needed to feminize a human embryo, essentially turning a baby boy (genetically predetermined) into a baby girl–is the same ratio as one drop of gin in 700 railway cars filled with tonic water.[29]

A tiny amount of toxin entering the body at a critical time in the body's development can produce a profound effect. However, it is the job of government and health officials to tell you not to worry…that everything will be fine. Some of these officials know the truth, yet they continue to advise you not to worry. But many of these same officials have no idea how serious the problem has become.

No one wants to face the true gravity and enormity of this issue. As mentioned earlier, our senses were not designed to detect things that do not belong here. It's no surprise that of all of the synthetic chemicals known, some of which cause disease, most are undetectable to our senses.

One of the ways that the U.S. government keeps track of and lists the toxins is by guidelines established by the Comprehensive Environmental Response, Compensation and Liability Act (CERCLA). This act requires the Agency for Toxic Substances and Disease Registry (ATSDR) and the EPA to prepare a list, in order of priority, of substances that are most commonly found at facilities on the National Priorities List (NPL) and which are determined to pose the most significant potential threat to human health due to their known or suspected toxicity and potential for human exposure at these NPL sites. CERCLA also requires this list to be revised periodically to reflect additional information on hazardous substances.

This CERCLA priority list is revised and published on a two-year basis, with a yearly informal review and revision. Each substance on the CERCLA Priority List of Hazardous Substances is a candidate to become the subject of a toxicological profile prepared by ATSDR and subsequently a candidate for the identification of priority data needs. This priority list is based on an algorithm that utilizes the following three components: frequency of occurrence at NPL sites, toxicity and potential for human exposure to the substances found at NPL sites. This algorithm utilizes data from ATSDR's HazDat database, which contains information from ATSDR's public health assessments and health consultations.

Having explained that, let's go back to the concept of hazardous and potentially deadly toxins being undetectable to human senses. One example would be the sixth most hazardous chemical on the CERCLA (2003) priority list–benzene. Breathing benzene can cause drowsiness, dizziness and unconsciousness; long-term benzene exposure produces harmful effects on the bone marrow and can cause anemia and leukemia. You cannot see benzene, but you can smell it. However, benzene becomes critically dangerous long before the concentrations are high enough for you to detect its scent or taste.

I discuss benzene several times in this book, but it is appropriate to serve as an example of how ill-equipped our senses are to detect toxins that do not belong on this planet. We cannot see them, taste them or smell them. Yet they are definitely present, and most of them (if not all of them) are already in us. If you have trouble with this fact, let's relate to something you know. You cannot see or smell oxygen in the air you breathe or the water you drink, but it is there nonetheless. Unlike chemical toxins, however, oxygen is life-giving, and you do not need to know it is there because without it there would be no life as we know it.

Most people can start to smell benzene in the air at 1.5–4.7 parts of benzene per million parts of air (ppm). They can smell benzene in water at 2 ppm. The EPA has set the maximum permissible level of benzene in drinking water at 5 parts per billion (ppb). One ppb is one 1000th of a ppm. Therefore, long before you can smell benzene, you will have already far exceeded safe levels. Most people can't begin to taste benzene in water until it reaches 0.5–4.5 ppm–again, far beyond safe levels.

Benzene is found in the air, water and soil. Because it can cause leukemia, the EPA has set a goal of 0 ppb for benzene in drinking water, in addition to water such as rivers and lakes. If the EPA and its sister agencies in other countries get the funding and legislation they need, I believe they can make this vitally needed change happen. The EPA recommends a maximum permissible level of benzene in water at 200 ppb for short-term exposures (10 days) for children. Their smaller bodies simply can't handle the same level of toxins as adults.

As I mentioned earlier, there are over 75,000 synthetic chemicals that have been introduced to our environment since 1930. Only about 7% of these have been tested for safety in adults and around 3% in children. This means that the toxicities of about 70,000 chemicals are simply unknown at this point. As we breathe and drink chemicals that adversely affect our immune systems, nervous systems and cognitive function, we remain totally unaware of them and assume we are symptom-free. We take in these toxins in such small amounts each day that we go on about our business thinking we're well. We believe if we see the sky is blue and the air looks clear, that in fact it must also be free of toxin.

While lecturing in Southern California, I was fortunate enough to have an extra day at a beachfront hotel. I couldn't see the danger in the ocean, but the beach was posted "closed." The sign also said, "Avoid water contact due to chemical contamination." Not an uncommon sight according to many beachfront residents in that area.

Far too infrequently we see mainstream media, designed for consumption by the general public, publishing useful information about the environment and its effects on human health. One such article was *National Wildlife* magazine's "Truth about Dioxin."[30] Another example is *Discover* magazine's article called "Toxic Wind."[31] This very fine article, written by Michael L. Brown, starts with the wisdom that, "A witch's brew of exotic chemicals is wafting from the factories and farms and tainting the air and water, fish and fowl, and you and me." In this article, Brown does an excellent job of illustrating how weather systems circulate toxins from points you would never expect, bringing it to the most remote locations on Earth. He points out in his article how pesticides being sprayed in the southeastern United States can be swept up in weather systems and may end up in the upper peninsula of Michigan or the province of Ontario in Canada.

If that wasn't dramatic enough, tests now confirm that insecticides used to combat malaria-bearing mosquitoes in the tropics have shown up in fish from Yukon lakes. Chemicals used on crops in Central and South America are absorbed into the bodies of polar bears off the Yukon's North Slope.

Many of the pollutants detected in Yukon fish belong to a group of synthetic chemicals called organochlorines, which includes PCBs, DDT, toxaphene and a variety of other substances.[32] They know this since pesticides (being synthetic chemicals) leave a very precise footprint. We can document when these chemicals were sold and used. *The wind ensures that whatever we create will be distributed to all parts of the globe.*

There is no place on Earth that is completely safe. It doesn't matter if you live in Tibet, Montana, the Yukon or Peru. It doesn't matter if you are near factories or farms. You can live at the North Pole or the South Pole or anywhere in-between and still be exposed to the same hazardous chemicals. Every minute. Every hour. Every day...

References

1. What you Need to know about Mercury in Fish and Shellfish. U.S. Dept of Health & Human Services and U.S. Environmental Protection Agency. *EPA-823-R-04-005.* March 2004. (www.cfsan.fda.gov/~dms/admehg3.html)
2. Encarta Encyclopedia: http://encarta.msn.com/
3. Jacob U. Pesticides in surface and coastal waters. World Wildlife Fund Briefing, July 1998: http://www.ngo.grida.no/wwfneap/Publication/pubframe.htm.
4. Ott WR, Roberts, JW. Everyday exposure to toxic pollutants. *Scientific American;* Feb 1998:86-91.
5. Moyers B, Jones S. Trade Secrets: *A Moyers Report.* Public Affairs Television Inc., 2001: http://pbs.org/tradesecrets/
6. Rall DP, Hogan MD, Huff JE, et al. Alternatives to using human experience in assessing health risks. *Ann Rev Pub Health* 1987; 8:355-385.
7. International Agency for Research of Cancer. IARC Monograph on the evaluation of carcinogenic risks to humans; Overall evaluations of carcinogenicity; Update of IARC Monograph, Vols 1-42, Supplement 7, Lyon, France, 1987.
8. U.S. Department of Health and Human Services: http://www.hhs.gov/
9. Agency for Toxic Substances and Disease Registry. *Public health statement for DDT, DDE, and DDD,* September, 2002. http://www.atsdr.cdc.gov/toxprofiles/ phs35.html
10. Garabant DH, Langholz B, Peters JM, Mach TM. DDT and related compounds and risk of pancreatic cancer. *J Natl Cancer Inst* 1992;84(10):764-771.
11. World Health Organization (WHO). DDT and its Derivatives--Environmental Effects. *Environmental Health,* Criteria 83, 1989.
12. Johnson WW, Finley MT. *Handbook of Acute Toxicity of Chemicals to Fish and Aquatic Invertebrates.* Resource Publication 137. U.S. Dept. of Interior, Fish and Wildlife Service. Washington, DC., 1980.
13. Matsumura F 1985. *Toxicology of Insecticides.* Second Edition. Plenum Press, New

York, NY, 1985.

14. Hudson RH, Tucker RK, Haegele K. *Handbook of Acute Toxicity of Pesticides to Wildlife.* Resource Publication 153. U.S. Dept. of Interior, Fish and Wildlife Service, Washington, D.C., 1984.

15. U.S. Environmental Protection Agency. Environmental Fate and Effects Division. Pesticide Environmental Fate One Line Summary: DDT. Washington, DC, 1989.

16. New York State Department of Health. *Health Advisories: Chemicals in Game and Sportfish.* 1999-2000. http://www.health.state.ny.us/nysdoh/fish/99fish.pdf

17. Dinham B. Pesticides: more sales, more trade–and more hazards? *Pesticides   News* No. 32, June 1996:16.

18. Environmental News Network. Environmental toxics linked to childhood behavior problems. *Great Lakes Directory,* October 29, 2001: http://www.greatlakesdirectory.org/zarticles/1029toxins.htm

19. Learning Disability Association of America. Top child health agencies urge testing to protect early brain development from toxins: One out of six affected. New York, Jan. 22, 2001 /PRNewswire: http://www.prnewswire.com/cgi-bin/stories.pl?ACCT=104&%20STORY=/www/story/01-22-2001/0001408422& EDATE

20. Rice DC. Parallels between attention deficit hyperactivity disorder and behavioral deficits produced by neurotoxic exposure in monkeys. *Environ Health Perspec.* 2000;108(Suppl 3):405-408.

21. Harding KL, Judah RD, Gant C. Outcome-based comparison of Ritalin versus food-supplement-treated children with AD/HD. *Altern Med Rev.* 2003;8(3):319-330.

22. Kidd PM. Attention deficit/hyperactivity disorder (ADHD) in children: rationale for its integrative management. *Altern Med Rev.* 2000;5(5):402-428.

23. Dengate, S. Order In The House (a national newsletter for parents, educators and behavior management specialists about Attention Deficit Hyperactivity Disorder (ADHD) and related topics: http://www.fedupwithfoodadditives.info/information/oith/index2.htm

24. Pearson H. Pollutants mature sperm prematurely. *Nature News Service*; MacMillan Magazines July 3, 2002 1:1-3.

25. World Resources Institute, United Nations Environment Programme, United Nations Development Programme, and the World Bank, *Pressures On Marine Biodiversity, Pollution And Sedimentation,* 1996-1997.

26. Guynup S. Mysterious Kenya flamingo die-offs tied to toxins, study says. *National Geographic Today,* November 8, 2002.

27. Park A. How safe is salmon? *Time* magazine, Aug. 11, 2003.

28. Holmes M. Gender bender: Chemicals threaten human reproduction. *British Columbia Environmental Network Report.* 1995;Vol. 6(3):15. http://www.bcen.bc.ca/bcerart/Vol6/genderbe.htm

29. Bouma K. A true horror story: pesticides' effects on hormones: Lake Apopka's infamous gender-bent alligators aren't only a freak of modern pollution. *Orlando Sentinel.* Orlando, Fla.:Feb 1, 1998, pg.16A.

30. Monks V. The truth about dioxin. *National Wildlife* magazine. August-September, 1994.

31. Brown, M. Toxic wind. *Discover.* November, 1987, Volume 8.

32. Chemical Contamination is a Worldwide Problem. *Yukon News*: Your Yukon (Column 53): (sponsored by Environment Canada). http://www.taiga.net/your Yukon/col053.html#top

Chapter 6
Toxins in Your Home

Does Your HOUSE Make YOU Sick?

Alarming news is part of America's daily information diet. There have, however, been insufficient news reports focused on toxins in the environment and the increase in diseases of all kinds. The relationship between the two is undeniable, yet the media hasn't yet devoted newspaper-selling, rating-grabber headlines to it because few members of the media have the academic qualifications or interest to research it. As a result, the story is still stuck in the back pages, and the public knows virtually nothing about this alarming situation.

For years, I've been telling doctors, the public and the media about the correlation between toxins and disease. I am not the first or the only environmentalist, but my approach and my background are unique. Until recently, mine has been a lonely voice, crying out in the wilderness, hoping that someone will hear my message. After nearly 17 years of lecturing and writing about this issue in my international newsletter, *The Nugent Report*, I began to receive some mainstream validation of my theories and concerns. In February, 1998, *Scientific American* published the story that desperately needed to be told–the story of "Everyday Exposure to Toxic Pollutants."[1]

According to the scientists who did the research, Wayne Ott (formerly of the EPA) and L.A. Wallace, the concentration of toxins inside your home is 5 to 10 times higher than it is outdoors.[1] This ratio directly correlates with the air volume available in an enclosed area and the characteristics of the toxins themselves. Before I discuss the findings in that report, let me give you a clear understanding of how this can happen.

Elsewhere in this book, I mention temperature inversion layers and how they work. Under perfect conditions, the barrier should be invisible. Across most of North America, this layer sits about 1,000 feet above ground level. The barrier's height depends on many factors, including the amount of heat that the ground beneath either reflects or absorbs. In Los Angeles, for instance, this barrier stays at about 1,000 feet year-round. Yet in Fairbanks, Alaska during the winter, its height is only about 30 feet.

A temperature inversion layer this close to the ground creates a distinct health hazard. The State of Alaska has actually told the public that there is a correlation between heart disease and air pollution in Fairbanks. This correlation occurs since the volume of clean air available to mix with pollutants such as carbon monoxide and benzene (a cancer-causing by-product of burning fuel) from automobile exhaust is limited to about 30 feet in the winter. That means that with every breath you take in Fairbanks during the winter, you get more toxins by volume of air than you get in a typical day in Los Angeles, where you have 1,000 feet of air volume to mix with the pollutants. However, Los Angeles has a very visible brown dome of pollution, and Alaska does not. Unfortunately, when it comes to toxins, air color is not always a reliable indicator. As discussed in Chapter 5, the majority of the dangerous toxins we breathe every day are those that you cannot see or even smell. What you can't see can definitely hurt you.

Having established that, let's talk about enclosed places–your home, your office, public places like stores and restaurants or, even worse, bars. In these enclosed environments, we're subjected to extreme levels of toxins, including chloramine gas, other toxic gases, many pesticides, formaldehyde gas, benzene and toxic metals, such as lead and cadmium. Many of the chemicals we are exposed to every day have been shown to cause cancer. Some cause asthma, allergies, fatigue and a long list of other symptoms you'll learn about in "The Solution" section of this book. Some are known to contribute to heart disease. There is also evidence of organ damage in infants as well as childhood cancers from toxins in carpet fibers.[1,2,3]

This story is one of the most important you will ever read, but you need to be aware that there are many special interest groups that don't want this information to reach you or the public in general. That's never stopped me before, so read on for the rest of the story.

Interest in the connection between toxins in the home and the skyrocketing rate of virtually every disease known, especially those that affect children, is quite recent. In fact, this interest is still limited to very small numbers of scientists. As you're aware, before anything can be done about any disease or condition, the cause must be identified. There must be a diagnosis before the doctor can write a prescription.

Those of you who are familiar with Newtonian Law might recall Newton's Third Law of Motion, "For every action, there is an equal and opposite reaction." Modern physicists now argue the validity of Newtonian law, but it certainly applies here. You cannot pollute the environment and not expect a consequence. Many people have heard the phrase "garbage in/garbage out." Well, the new saying for our health should be "toxin in/disease out." When you wonder why children are falling victim to cancer, organ damage, allergies and asthma in ever-increasing numbers, you might look for the causes in your home first–in fact, right under your feet. (Wait until you learn the facts on childhood asthma in Chapter 12.)

Should we rely on the government to uncover these causes? Or does the responsibility belong to each of us? There are several schools of thought on this matter. I think after reading this far, you can already anticipate my thoughts.

Some people believe that the government automatically knows about all the problems that exist and will automatically correct them without any citizen having to worry about who will take care of the problem. People who think that way need a reality check. At the other end of the spectrum are those who believe that the government either will deliberately do nothing about problems or is continuously involved in conspiracies or subversive activities that are intended to undermine the citizens' well-being.

Of course, neither of these extreme points of view is completely accurate. There are politicians and appointed officials who lack the courage to tackle these issues, but more frequently it is a case of ignorance or worse–arrogance. You're no doubt familiar with the attitude that is so often characteristic of government officials: "I know all the issues. You are just a poor, dumb citizen, so don't try to confuse me with facts."

There are dedicated people in government too, people who aren't arrogant and try not to be ignorant. These people do what they can with the meager resources they have accessible. However, they are typically hampered in their efforts by greedy, self-serving politicians who don't want to appropriate money for anything that won't result in their staying in office.

Here's an example of what just a few conscientious people can accomplish:

The U.S. Environmental Protection Agency actually developed a method for testing indoor toxins in 1980. It was called Total Exposure Assessment Methodology or TEAM.

Using TEAM, the EPA group began as a government research project in 1985 to test exposure to everyday toxins. This project was called the Non-Occupational Pesticide Exposure Study (NOPES) and was conducted by Wayne Ott and L. A. Wallace.

Initial research was conducted primarily by the Triangle Institute, a research group in North Carolina.[2] As the study progressed, it expanded to include two dozen other contract research organizations in 14 states. In addition, money was provided by private industry to fund studies in Alaska as well as one Canadian province.

One of the study groups looked only for the presence of DDT. As I mentioned earlier, while DDT has been illegal for use in the U.S. since 1972, oddly enough this country remains the world's largest manufacturer of that terrible toxin. The U.S. allows the sale of DDT to any country that wants to buy it, and the chemical's pervasive nature sends it back to us by way of the air or in the water.

The chemical name for DDT is dichlorodiphenyltrichloroethane. (Now you can understand why everyone, including scientists, just says DDT.) Jonathan D. Buckley, a researcher at the University of Southern California, and David E. Camann, of Southwest Research Institute, found that 90 of the 362 midwestern homes they examined in 1992 and 1993 had DDT in the carpets, despite the fact that it had been illegal for use in the United States for 20 years.[1,2] **In more than half of the households that Buckley and Camann surveyed, the concentrations of seven toxic organic chemicals, called polycyclic aromatic hydrocarbons–compounds which are known to cause cancer in animals and are thought to induce cancer in humans–were above the levels that would trigger a formal risk assessment at a federally funded Superfund site.**

Concentrations of Pesticides[1]

The blue bars on the pesticide chart (Plate 4) represent the indoor levels of various pesticides. The yellow bars represent the outdoor levels of those same pesticides, where they were originally sprayed. The scientific team tested homes totally at random in the both the U.S. and Canada. The same patterns appeared wherever they tested.

In order to be effective, pesticides must not only be able to kill insects. They must also be sticky. They have to stick to leaves, fruit and vegetables. This same stickiness causes them to stick to the bottoms of our shoes. As we walk indoors, we take these chemicals from the bottom of our shoes and deposit them in our carpets. The scientists found that the deeper the carpets, the greater the percentage of pesticides and other toxins found. Deep shag carpets had more toxin than short nap carpets. In addition, they found other toxins like lead in the carpeting. It's simple–the deeper the pile, the worse the problem is.

(I understand that shag, which has been out of fashion for some years, is coming back now but under a new name. My recommendation is to avoid shag by any name. In fact, I would avoid carpet wherever I could. Most of my own home has non-porous surfaces including wood, marble or granite floors).

Pesticides and volatile organic chemicals found indoors have been confirmed to cause at least 3,000 cases of cancer each year in the U.S. alone, making these substances just as dangerous as radon gas. Keep in mind that the overwhelming number of cancer patients are never screened for the cause of their cancers. This is particularly true of testing for toxins. In my opinion, if every cancer patient were screened for toxins, the number of cases confirmed to be caused by toxins would soar dramatically into the tens of thousands per year!

Finding this concentration of toxins came as a surprise to almost all researchers, especially since DDT has been banned since 1972 in the U.S. and Canada. Nevertheless, it's still found in our homes. Jonathan D. Buckley of the University of Southern California and David E. Camann of the Southwest Research Institute found that 90 of the 362 Midwestern homes they examined in 1992 and 1993 had DDT in the carpets.[1,2]

The presence of DDT puts everyone in the home at risk, especially any family member who spends time on the floor–which, of course, means our very young children. Any toxins that do not biodegrade will simply continue to spread around the world and contribute to poor health of the planet. Many dangerous toxins (apparently not all) will break down over time if exposed to sufficient sunlight, air and or water; these conditions do not exist in our homes. So the toxins not only linger they accumulate. There is no place on Earth that does not have some level of toxins. But what scientists found in our homes is truly shocking.

More unseen threats

This is just the tip of the toxic iceberg. Another study tested 178 homes for any form of toxin. It produced results more alarming than anyone imagined. The purpose of the tests was to determine the presence of volatile organic compounds, or VOCs, as well as respirable particles, or RPs. Volunteers were designated in each home that agreed to be tested (Plate 5). They agreed to wear or carry special monitoring devices throughout normal daily activities.[1]

Altogether, 3,000 people took part in the various tests. They represented a broad enough study base to make the results impossible to ignore. In studying the test results, many of the researchers were surprised to find that the indoor levels of toxins were far higher than the outdoor levels. This was even true in the cities of Bayonne and Elizabeth in New Jersey, where toxic chemicals produced by industry reach some of their highest levels in North America. Even in those two highly polluted cities, tests still found that measurements of 11 VOCs were higher indoors than they were outdoors.

To illustrate the unanticipated effects of chemicals, let's look at benzene, a chemical known to cause leukemia in workers exposed to high concentrations. Benzene is a by-product of gasoline found primarily in automobile exhaust. It is also found in other fuels, such as jet aircraft fuel. However, it's also one of the 4,000 toxic chemicals found in tobacco smoke. While you don't inhale automobile exhaust on a regular basis, living with a smoker raises your exposure to benzene significantly.

In 1985, Dr. Wallace compiled information on several hundred people living in five different states and how they were exposed to benzene. His findings indicated that the average concentration of benzene being inhaled was three times higher indoors than the typical outdoor levels. His calculations showed that 45% of the U.S. population's total exposure to benzene comes from cigarette smoking, 36% from inhaling gasoline fumes and using other common products such as glues, and 16% from sources such as paints stored in the home.[3] *It seems clear from Wallace's work that indoor pollution appears to pose a far greater health risk to people than outdoor pollution.*

Most people, including some government officials and many individuals in the media, persist in believing that the majority of toxins are outdoors, and that toxins can always be seen or smelled. That's why most measurement systems were developed to measure outdoor toxins only. Wallace's work demonstrates for us that reducing industrial emissions of benzene, for example, would have a very small impact on health in general. On the other hand, reducing cigarette smoking would have a major impact on the general health of the U.S., simply because of the reduction in exposure to benzene.

Since benzene is known to cause cancer in laboratory animals and leukemia in humans, it follows that reducing benzene exposure would reduce the statistical occurrence of leukemia at the least. According to Michael McCally, MD, PhD, Mount Sinai School of Medicine, **"Current normal body burdens of dioxin and several other well-studied organochlorines in humans are at or near the range at which toxic effects occur in laboratory animals."**[4] Dr. McCally has been doing continuing research in the area of toxins and their effects on human health. He has discovered virtually every patient tested has toxic body burdens.

As mentioned in a previous chapter, former U.S. Assistant Surgeon General David Rall has said, "Every chemical known to cause cancer in humans also causes cancer in experimental animals. While some species are more sensitive to toxic effects than others, laboratory studies have proved to be good predictors of health effects in humans." No, I didn't get that backwards–he was making a very important point by that very deliberate choice of words. So for those who say well it only kills lab animals, but is yet to be proven in humans, take a deep breath and think about what Dr. Rall said.

The Dietary Supplement Health and Education Act (DSHEA) of 1994 in the U.S. requires that only scientifically studied and published material be discussed as fact. That's as it should be. However, this constraint often precludes some common sense observations. I mentioned that reducing cigarette smoking in the U.S. would have a significant impact on health because that's what was studied. But clearly people worldwide are affected adversely by benzene and other toxins in cigarettes, and that's of significance as well.

Your home contains more than one threat to your health. Scientists have discovered that there are toxins of various types throughout the house. As an example, you have toxins in your closet. If you are like most Americans, you have some clothing in your closet that has been dry cleaned. Dry cleaners use a fluid that they call "perc," which is tetrachloroethylene, also known as perchloroethylene. Perc has been found to cause cancer in laboratory animals and is suspected of causing cancer in humans. Think about what Dr. Rall said.

There may be other cancer-causing agents in your closet, as well. Have you ever wondered why a moth won't go near a mothball? Perhaps the moth knows something we don't know. Most moth crystals in mothballs contain a chemical known as paradichlorobenzene, which causes cancer in laboratory animals. This chemical, by the way, has also been used in toilet disinfectants. Clean and aesthetically pleasing toilets are important but not at the cost of attacking your immune system and possibly inviting cancer. The old-fashioned method is still best in this area. How badly do you need blue toilet water?

(In chapter 11, I'll give you some natural recipes to replace most of the toxins discussed in this chapter).

Then there's formaldehyde and styrene gas from dry ink toners, most notably copy machines. "Formaldehyde is also found in glues for wallpapers and surfacing materials like counter tops. (Formaldehyde) causes cancer, induces asthma, allergies, headaches and fatigue."[1] Plate 6 shows sources of toxins in homes and offices that will surprise many.

We are even exposed to toxins when we take a shower in the morning! That's not just because of the toxins in the water itself. In most municipal water systems, the water is cleaned with chlorine. But every morning, when you take a hot shower and heat that water to a steam, you are producing chloramine gas. We only get small amounts of the chloramine gas as we shower each day, but it's still not a very healthful activity. To diminish the effect, it's important to have a well-ventilated area for showering so that the gas can rise away from you. The process is somewhat like the inversion layer concept I introduced at the beginning of this chapter.

Another substance that has been studied recently is carbon monoxide. Although new U.S. standards have resulted in cleaner automobile exhaust and a decrease in carbon monoxide levels, we clearly have a higher level of carbon monoxide inside our homes that is not affected by these new federal standards. While carbon monoxide isn't good for any of us, it's particularly dangerous to individuals with poor circulation or heart problems, and, unfortunately, the number of people with poor cardiovascular health is growing. Governments have focused on measuring toxins outdoors but the greater threats to us as individuals remain largely recognized. Scientists like Wayne Ott are trying to change that.[5]

Another area of recent research has investigated respirable particles, or RPs. In the study of 178 homes in Riverside, California mentioned earlier in this section, volunteers carried devices that gathered particles small enough to penetrate into the lungs–those that are ten microns in diameter or smaller.[1] Concurrent air samples taken indoors and outdoors showed that exposure from particulate levels indoors during the day were about 60% greater than expected. This increase occurred because we stir up these particles as we move around the house.

Picture a nice, sunny day when you've walked around your house and watched particles of dust floating through rays of sunlight in front of you. Ott and Roberts refer to this as your personal toxic dust cloud. That's a fairly common experience. Sadly, many of those particles are RPs containing toxins that can penetrate your lungs and cause a potential threat to your health–potentially even a free radical disease. Recent epidemiological studies have associated an elevated concentration of RPs outdoors with premature death. RPs may, in fact, be hastening the aging process. The breakdown of cells triggered by RPs occurs at a rate faster than nature intended. And the levels of RPs indoors are far greater than outdoors.

Volatile Organic Compounds[1]
Perhaps more disturbing news comes from two other studies of indoor air contaminants conducted during the late 1980s in Jacksonville, Florida and Springfield, Massachusetts.[2]

These studies revealed that indoor air contained a concentration of pesticides at least five times higher (more typically ten times higher) than the outside air. Those residues included insecticides approved only for outdoor use. Ott and Roberts point out in their excellent article in the February 1998 issue of *Scientific American* that most of these contaminants are tracked in on our shoes.[1] They may also seep through the soil into our homes in the form of a gas. For example, chlordane was removed from the list of products sold for home use in 1988, yet it was still showing up in tests inside homes more than 10 years later. Please take a look at color plate 5 near the center of the book to see a chart of Volatile Organic Compounds or VOC's measured in homes. You'll note many unfamiliar chemicals that are difficult to pronounce. The rule I use to give my patients is,

"If you can't pronounce it don't eat it." Yet is seems we are eating these things whether we like it or not.

Other pesticides contaminating indoor air are also exposing residents to higher rates of those substances than are found in food. These pesticides, which are broken down by sunlight and bacteria over just a few days outdoors, can last for several years in indoor carpets, where, according to Ott, they're protected from these same elements.

TOXINS IN YOUR HOME[1]

Everyday toxins: You're better off outdoors.

Your children are at the highest risk!

Have you ever heard the phrase "cancer clusters?" The first time anyone used this term was a few years after atomic testing had been conducted in Nevada. Clusters of people, especially children, were all being diagnosed with the same cancer at the same time. Cancer is not contagious, so how could this happen?

Simple: All the cancer victims had been exposed to radiation from the atomic bomb tests at the same time, resulting in the same problem occurring in clusters. Now we hear that term used particularly when many children of approximately the same age contract the same cancer in the same city area. This condition occurs because they are all exposed to the same cancer-causing toxic chemical at the same time and in an amount that their small bodies simply cannot tolerate. That is why it takes years longer for an adult to get the same cancer from that toxin.

We shouldn't see the presence of cancer in children at all, especially not in infants. However, children are getting more cancer-causing toxins in their bodies today than adults. Read on and you will understand why.

During the last five years of my medical practice, I saw an ever-increasing number of infants and children with ailments and diseases that infants and children should not have, especially in such progressively increasing numbers. I consulted several of my colleagues who confirmed that they, too, were seeing unusual increases in children and infants with ailments that we should not have been seeing, especially in such high numbers.

Infants are particularly susceptible to organ damage when exposed to various volatile organic compounds and RPs. Because of their low body weight, their risk per pound is significantly multiplied when they ingest the same amount of toxic dust that adults do. Because they spend much of their time on the floor, primarily on carpets, it is estimated that the average infant ingests 100 milligrams of toxic chemicals every day. According to Ott and Roberts, we can now estimate that each day the average urban infant will ingest 110 nanograms of benzo(a)pyrene, the most toxic polycyclic aromatic hydrocarbon known. This is equivalent to the child's smoking three cigarettes a day, and at a child's body weight, that is a devastatingly high amount.[1,6] For small children, house dust is also a major source of toxic metals, such as cadmium, lead and possibly other heavy metals. It is also a source of polychlorinated biphenyls or PCBs, which were shown in a Wayne State University study to lower IQ in children.

Carpets are the culprits. They act as reservoirs for these toxic compounds in addition to dangerous bacteria, asthma-inducing allergens and toxic metals. The deeper the pile, the more likely that toxins are there; the shorter the pile, the safer the carpet. If the surfaces are completely smooth, as are wood and tile floors, you have the lowest possible risk of accumulating toxins and the strongest possibility of being able to clean any throw rugs thoroughly.

Roberts, one of the scientists who contributed to the report published in the February 1998 issue of *Scientific American*, and several other colleagues showed that one could prevent the accumulation of dangerous amounts of toxic dust by using a vacuum equipped to sense that there are no more particles to be extracted. As far as I know, these vacuums are not yet available for general use, but they make a strong case for using the highest quality vacuum cleaner available.

In another study, researchers found that merely wiping your feet on an industry-standard doormat could reduce the amount of toxin in the carpets by a factor of six. Although this is a very significant result, don't be fooled into thinking that wiping your feet will eliminate the danger entirely.

Lead exposure from paint has nearly been eliminated in most U.S. cities, but it is still being found in carpets. Confirmed to reduce IQ in humans, lead exposure is thought to affect more than 900,000 children in the U.S. currently.[1] Therefore, the simple act of using good doormats would translate to a meaningful increase in public health and IQ in children. Or we could choose to remove our shoes, as the Japanese and other Far East cultures do. That's perhaps the easiest, most intelligent first step to take.

(I will give you more details on lead in Chapter 12).

As the presence of toxins increases, the time we are exposed to them also increases. The rates of diseases are also on the rise–particularly exotic diseases, autoimmune diseases, neuromuscular diseases and new diseases being diagnosed with greater frequency now than in the past. These toxic chemicals are not natural to our planet, or anywhere else for that matter. They do not belong here. The human body was not designed to encounter or defend itself from these chemicals. Therefore, we live in a time when we have no choice but to take extraordinary measures to protect ourselves. This is the 21st century. We have changed our world, and now we must change the ways we look at health care as well as the ways we care for our world.

In summary, the threats from toxins in your home are at least five, and more frequently ten, times higher than they are outdoors. These threats include chemicals that are known to cause cancer, lower immune function and IQ, and induce asthma, allergies, headaches and fatigue. Some of these chemicals may also affect the nervous system and even your ability to think clearly and pay attention. In "The Solution" section of this book, I will discuss some of the things you can do to improve the safety of your home and the health of your family as it relates to toxins there.

Once again, do not deceive yourself: Just because you cannot see, smell or taste these chemicals, it is a mistake to think that you're healthy just because you feel fine. Today, in the 21st century, how you feel is simply no longer an accurate gauge of your health and most of the greatest threats are chemicals you cannot detect with your senses.

References and further reading
1. Ott WR, Roberts JW. Everyday exposure to toxic pollutants. *Scientific American.* February 1998:86-91.
2. Whitmore RW, Immerman FW, Camann DE, et al. Non-occupational exposure to

pesticides for residents of two U.S. cities. *Arch Environ Contam Toxicol* 1994;26(1): 47-59.

3. Wallace LA. Human exposure to environmental pollutants: a decade of experience. *Clin Exp Allergy* 1995;25(1):4-9.

4. Moyers B, Jones S. Trade Secrets: A Moyers Report. Public Affairs Television Inc., 2001: http://www.pbs.org/tradesecrets/

5. Ott WR. Human exposure assessment: The birth of a new science. *J Exposure Anal Environ Epidemiol* 1995;5(4):449-472.

6. Roberts JW, Dickey P. Exposure of children to pollutants in house dust and indoor air. *Revs Environ Contamin Toxicol* 1995;143:59-78.

Chapter 7
Drugs in the drinking Water

The unfortunate truth is that we all take drugs.

More than 100 published reports done on drinking water in cities all over the world confirm that we get pharmaceutical drugs in our water every day.[1] This information is so new (and disturbing) that the media hasn't gotten hold of it yet and virtually no doctors are aware of it, let alone the public.

This news is alarming for many reasons. First, according to statistics published in the *Journal of the American Medical Association* (JAMA), adverse reactions to FDA-approved, double-blind-tested prescription drugs are the fourth-leading cause of death in the USA.[2] All you have to do is look up any drug in the massive *Physician's Desk Reference* for drugs and read the millions of words that warn of side effects and adverse reactions, sometimes including death. You know you don't want to take these drugs unless it is absolutely necessary for your health. However, you apparently have no choice.

To put the health statistics in perspective and to answer your inevitable questions on what are the other causes of death and how many, I have included two charts below.

First let's look at the leading causes of death according to the Centers for Disease Control and Prevention (CDC) then we'll look at the reality of how pharmaceutical drugs affect our population. I have listed the official top ten causes of death in the U.S. so you can see just how serious this pharmaceutical drug issue is. Since pharmaceuticals that are properly prescribed kill more than 100,000 American every year. it is a very serious health issue that gets far too little attention from government health officials.

Number of deaths for leading causes of death[3] (Data are for U.S. in 2001)

1. Heart disease	700,142
2. Cancer	553,768
3. Stroke	163,538
4. Chronic lower respiratory diseases	123,013
5. Accidents (unintentional injuries)	101,537
6. Diabetes	71,372
7. Influenza/pneumonia	62,034
8. Alzheimer's disease	53,852
9. Nephritis, nephrotic syndrome and nephrosis	39,480
10. Septicemia	32,238

Leading Causes of Death
Adverse reactions to prescription drugs are the fourth-largest cause of death nationally.[2]

1. Heart disease:	700,142[4]
- One of every 2 people will experience heart disease.	
- In 50% of the cases, the first symptom is death.	
2. Cancer:	553,768[5]
- In 1971, cancer was the 7th-leading cause of death.	
- Cancer is predicted to increase by more than 70% by 2010.	
3. Medical mistakes, infections and pharmaceutical drugs:	225,000[6]
– 106,000 non-error negative effects	
– 80,000 infections in hospitals	
– 20,000 other errors in hospitals of drugs[2]	
– 12,000 unnecessary surgeries	
– 7,000 medication errors in hospitals	
Total of medically induced deaths:	**225,000**

The first studies in this area were conducted as a result of an accidental discovery. (That's not an unusual occurrence in science.) Scientists in Berlin were searching for pesticide residue in drinking water–a monthly routine check. They found a chemical that had similarities to a pesticide, but it wasn't anything they recognized. They sent the sample to a lab, and it was identified as clofibric acid.[7] This is the generic name for a common drug prescribed to lower cholesterol.

The researchers were amazed and shocked! Nobody had ever considered this possibility before. Most people have faith that the water coming out of their tap is clean and safe. These same researchers then checked ground water and again found clofibric acid.[7]

Tests of both city tap water and well water confirm that we do not utilize all of the drugs we take. What our bodies do not utilize returns to the water table eventually via urine and/or feces. It then goes to a waste treatment plant that is reasonably, but not absolutely, equipped to remove bacteria, virus and many toxic chemicals–but not drugs. Since drugs are synthetics, they apparently remain intact and will not biodegrade. At this point, there is no way to know just how long they may remain intact as drugs in our drinking water before they will break down, if ever.

For several years, scientists have been speculating on the reason why so many common bacteria are becoming resistant to drugs. A common misperception is that this resistance is due strictly to over-prescribing by physicians. It is true that many doctors do prescribe antibiotics for viral infections, knowing full well that they will not affect the virus since antibiotics kill only bacteria.

In Canada, a survey showed that about 65% of Canadian doctors prescribe antibiotics for viral infections. They do so, as do American doctors, because a bacterial infection may ensue as a virus compromises the immune system. Many doctors prescribe antibiotics without knowing for certain if the medication they are prescribing is right for the bacteria in question because they do not do a culture to analyze which bacteria the patient has, and therefore which antibiotic would be most effective. The attitude is that if the first one doesn't work, just prescribe another, different one.

This is not the reason that bacteria are becoming increasingly resistant to antibiotics, however. *The main reason is that antibiotics are in our tap and well drinking water as well as much of our food.* According to Dr. Stuart Levy, Director of the Center for Adaptation Genetics and Drug Resistance at Tufts University in Boston, "Our concentration of antibiotics is 1,000 times higher than in the German drinking water. High enough to affect the growth of *E-coli* bacteria. This may be causing the bacteria to become medication-resistant."[8] In this quote, Dr. Levy was referring to the early studies cited above that found drugs in the Berlin drinking water. When he said, "our drinking water," he meant U.S. drinking water.

Some bacteria are now immune to even our most powerful antibiotics. That's a frightening prospect by any standard. This time science cannot come to the rescue. I will tell you in "The Solution" section of this book about the greatest hope for the human immune system. First, however, I must continue with the rest of this story.

The Berlin research team I mentioned also found other lipid- (fat-) lowering drugs, as well as analgesics (pain killers, including ibuprofen), chemotherapy drugs, antibiotics and hormones in tap water. A researcher, Thomas Ternes, found all of the above-mentioned drugs, plus thirty more antibiotics, beta-blockers, anti-seizure medication, and contrast agents for x-rays.[9]

Source of the Problems

Why are we seeing a worldwide increase of genetic disease? According to a scientist named Andreas Hartman, "…a class of broad-spectrum antibiotics in drinking water is causing toxicity to human DNA!"[10] Could this be a factor in the Parkinson's disease now thought by researchers not to be caused by genetics as mentioned earlier?

What about the widely published information that indicates a feminizing of living creatures and perhaps human males on this planet?[11] I wrote about this issue in 1995, and then again in 1997, in *The Nugent Report*. At that time, nobody wanted to believe me, and the majority asked if I could prove in every instance what the source of the feminizing chemicals was. At the time, I could prove only a few, but now the evidence has become all too clear.

Estrogen-like chemicals are rampant in our environment. They are also sometimes called endocrine (glandular) disruptors (EDs). These chemicals include the all-too-familiar PCBs (polychlorinated biphenyls and dioxins), and the not-so-familiar DDEs (a metabolite of DDT). Recall that earlier I spoke of a newspaper article in which Louis Guillete, a reproductive biologist from the University of Florida, positively confirmed what I had theorized years earlier. He was talking about xenoestrogens like dioxin, PCBs and DDE. But the results are the same in terms of feminizing effects, whether the cause is dioxin or birth control pills.[8]

These feminizing chemicals such as DDT, dioxins and dozens of other chemicals trick the body into thinking they are hormones. Those who don't want to face this unsettling reality of our age believe that there aren't enough toxins to make a difference. However, you may recall from an earlier chapter that Guillete put an end to that nonsense when he stated that, "The amount of estrogen needed to feminize a human embryo–essentially turning a baby boy into a baby girl–is the same ratio as one drop of gin in 700 railway cars full of tonic water."

You don't have to be a scientist to figure out that every tiny bit of toxin in our water affects our health!

A researcher from Michigan State University named Shane Snyder went to Lake Mead in Nevada, which is the primary water source for that entire region. He studied the fish in Lake Mead and conducted the same test 30 times to ensure that his data was correct. He found that the level of estrogen–not xenoestrogens like dioxin or PCBs, but pharmaceutical estrogen like birth control pills–was so high in Lake Mead that male fish were producing female egg protein.[12] Common sense tells us that male fish shouldn't be doing that. However neither we nor other animals now live on the type of planet we were designed to live on.

Two facts become abundantly clear from this information: First, we must start doing everything we can to remove these toxic drugs from our systems and learn how to maintain balance in our immune and hormone systems in view of this newly discovered threat to our health. Second, we must find a way to make our immune systems strong enough to resist medication-resistant bacteria since we can no longer rely on drugs in every case to save us if we get a bacterial infection. It is unfortunate, but based on current trends, the day will come when antibiotics will be of no use at all, and we will have to rely solely on our own immune systems to protect us. Our bodies can only do that if they have the proper fuel or tools to do that job. *Food alone can no longer provide us with the nutrition our bodies need to fight the ravages of today's environment. Dietary supplements are now a necessity!*

(It's very understandable if you feel uncomfortable at this point in the book. This kind of information should make everyone uncomfortable. However, I want to assure you that there is hope!)

Looking Back to See the Future

Let's go back in history to the middle 1300s when the most infamous of the black plagues occurred in Europe. Bubonic plague spread like wildfire across the European continent in the 1340s. Most scholars agree that one-third of the population of Europe died during the plague years. Most historians agree on a figure of approximately 25 million people. They also agree that *virtually everyone was exposed to the bubonic plague* during that period of time. This general exposure was due to horrendously filthy living conditions where whole families spent their entire lives dwelling in the same room. Sanitary conditions were generally non-existent, and it was virtually impossible to avoid exposure to microbes.

What's interesting is that the entire population was exposed, but only one-third of the population died from the bubonic plague. This tells us that a substantial number of Europeans had immune systems strong enough to resist and survive this onslaught. In "The Solution" section of this book I'll discuss the nutrients that support immune function, which are vitally important today. These nutrients are even more important now than they were in the 1340s.

Generally, most people believe that the bubonic plague and other epidemics are a thing of the past. However, this isn't the case. In the late 20th century, there was an outbreak of bubonic plague in India that fortunately was contained in that nation. In 2003, scientists discovered that there were squirrels carrying bubonic

plague on the California side of Lake Tahoe. This was cause for alarm, and this situation is being tracked very carefully at this point.

The real danger is that we have bacteria, which can slowly but certainly become resistant to antibiotics. We also have viruses that have mutated, such as the AIDS virus. Our immune system can't deal with them at all. It is more important than ever before that our immune system functions at absolutely optimal level at all times.

Increasing numbers of viruses, often previously unknown to the human population, are being released from rain forests as we deforest them. With very rapid international travel today, a person can go almost anywhere in the world in a number of hours. It is too easy for someone who has contracted a virus or bacteria–someone who doesn't have symptoms yet since they may take several days to appear–to get on a plane, fly to another city, expose everyone on the plane, and expose everyone they meet at airports, hotels, etc. Before you know it, an illness or disease will spread rapidly–perhaps exponentially.

Experts in the study of influenza viruses are very concerned. They tell us that influenza pandemics–epidemics that occur around the world–happen at regular intervals. They say that we are presently overdue for another pandemic, similar to the so-called "Spanish flu" that killed about 20 million people worldwide in 1918-19. I say "so-called" Spanish flu because like all flus and the black plague of the 1340s, they originated in Western China, not Spain. They also predict that as many as 60 million people may die in the next flu pandemic. Clearly, ensuring that our immune systems are as strong as they can possibly be, and working on ways to improve our environmental conditions, is of paramount importance to everyone everywhere.

Medication-resistant bacteria, of course, have become extremely common. Reports about them appear in newspapers, on TV and on radio frequently.

You may recall an article from *Time* magazine called "Killer Bacteria," which reported that *E. coli* bacteria was coming out of people's tap water in Wyoming.[13] Health officials were surprised, but told us not to worry. They said the same thing could never happen again. However, it did happen again in Ontario province in Canada. What was very significant about this was NOT that it was *E. coli* bacteria. (That's serious enough.) This was a new breed of *medication-resistant E. coli*.

Today, the use of antibiotics is more frequent in the United States than in any other industrialized nation. But antibiotics are being used worldwide. Moreover, some antibiotics now have become almost totally useless in the fight against bacteria. Many patients who are told to take the antibiotics for a given number of days have certainly misused them. They stop when their symptoms stop because they, of course, don't want to take pharmaceutical drugs. However, this tends to cause the bacteria that survive to become resistant to future courses of that antibiotic. So, patients share some of the blame too. If your doctor orders you to take a particular antibiotic for a particular number of days, follow doctor's orders!

At this point, there is still no known third-party, objectively validated filtration method that that has been shown to remove all pharmaceutical drugs from drinking water. (Before you jump to any hasty conclusions, please read this entire section.) I'm not saying that such a device does not exist. I'm simply saying that I have not seen any objective third-party data verifying, scientifically, that there is a device that can do this.

After publishing the first edition of this book, I received hundreds of contacts from people who were convinced that they had a water filtration system that could remove pharmaceuticals. After spending a great deal of time examining all these systems and their claims, I found myself back on square one–no systems I have yet seen can do this. Please re-examine the advertising, sales information and system directions from whatever company you may have purchased from or perhaps that you represent as a sales person. Most of the filtration devices I have thus far examined have produced very cleverly worded marketing materials that mislead people into thinking their water systems can do more than they have been scientifically proven to do.

Of course, there are also companies that claim to manufacture devices that can filter out virtually every type of toxin imaginable. Although some companies have tested for hundreds of toxins, none have tested in controlled tests through a third-party lab for the more than 75,000 synthetics and thousands of pharmaceutical drugs, plus all the volatile organics.

The idea that we are all taking virtually every known drug each time we drink water is pretty darn scary. Thus far in all communities tested, many (but not all) categories of the drugs present are not screened. There are thousands of drugs, and most water filtration companies don't even realize that there are drugs present in our drinking water, so of course they are not testing for them.

Let's take this concept one mind-boggling step further: Since drugs have been detected in the drinking water of more than 100 cities, it is safe to assume they are widespread. However, since tests have not revealed all known drugs, it is possible certain drugs that, for example, combine with chlorine and create a totally new compound, are as yet unknown. So just what should we be testing for? The thought of all the endless combinations and compounds that could theoretically result from these combinations is beyond comprehension! So, objectively speaking, there is never likely to be anything out there that is third-party-certified to remove all toxins. What I call the "compound-combining effect" will be explored in Chapter 13, and the conclusions we will have to draw are far more frightening to me than even the pharmaceutical issue. This information will really shock you too!

Many companies–especially those that sell reverse osmosis (RO) filtration systems–are supremely overconfident in their product despite the fact they have no evidence about drugs specifically. (RO systems will also be discussed in Chapter 13.) **So once again, it is not that there isn't a system that is capable of doing this. I believe there probably is, but it is my duty to be objective, and there is a distinct difference between desire or belief and the proven facts.**

What I have found is a number of filtration systems that do a good job, typically filtering at least 98% of bacteria, chlorine, many parasites and metals, as well as pesticides and chemicals of various types. But these systems do not filter pharmaceuticals yet for the reasons stated above.

Beyond the pharmaceutical issue, the key question these days is how healthful and natural is the water once it has completed the filtration process? Life is dependent on water, and it needs to be as natural as possible. In chapter 13, you will learn that sometimes filtration methods, while thorough in toxin removal, may result in less than healthy water.

I must re-emphasize that antibiotics are being put in drinking water around the world, and as a result, everyone drinks a small amount of antibiotic in their water each day. This not only has an adverse effect on your intestinal flora–essential for colon health, immune function, hormonal function and digestive function–but over time also tends to make these bacteria resistant to medication.

"In some communities, up to 40 percent of pneumococcal infections have become RESISTANT to a variety of antibiotics."

– U.S. News and World Report, May 1999[14]

Antibiotics are overused in animals, as well. Many animals are fed antibiotics, either because they are ill or, in the worst-case scenario, because they might someday become ill. Traces of these antibiotics are then consumed by humans in various meat products, eggs and dairy products. Of course, this amount of antibiotic taken into our bodies also compromises our immune function and can use our bodies as an incubator to cause bacteria to become more medication-resistant each year.

Rising Resistance
- *S. aureus* (Staph) is 32% resistant vs. methicillin.
- *S. aureus* (Staph) is 98% resistant vs. penicillin.
- *E. faecium* is 70% resistant vs. ciprofloxian (Cipro).
- *E. faecium* is 70% resistant vs. ampicillin.
- *S. pneumoniae* (strep) is 10% resistant vs. tetracycline.
- *S. pneumoniae* (strep) is 37% resistant vs. penicillin.

– Scientific American, March 1998[15]

The oldest antibiotic, penicillin, is now almost completely useless against staphylococcus bacteria. Over time, this alarming trend will continue with all antibiotics. This is why we must now take action ourselves to make our immune systems as strong as we can. Antibiotics in food and water now make a probiotic dietary supplement a necessity daily. Probiotic means the friendly, healthy flora needed by the human intestines. We'll discuss that further in coming chapters.

Conclusions
The ultimate effects of the numerous pharmaceuticals in drinking water are yet unknown. We all drink minute amounts of virtually every drug daily, and what effects if any they will have on us I do not know. *But we do know* several very important facts:

- We know that in some cases antibiotics in drinking water have already contributed to the growing rates of antibiotic-resistant bacteria (remember our earlier discussion of *E. coli*).

- We know that pharmaceuticals are unhealthful for the sensitive balance of microflora in our intestines.

- And we certainly know the dangers of chlorine and that heating chorinated water increases our health risks up to and including cancers.

In today's world, we cannot live without chlorine, but we cannot live long with it either. At the bare minimum, you must–I repeat, <u>**you must**</u>–have a filtration device that removes chlorine from your drinking and bathing water. (See more details on chlorine and the compound-combining effect in chapter 13.)

References
1. Halling-Serensen B, et al. Occurrence, fate and effects of pharmaceutical substances in the environment–a review. *Chemosphere* 1998;36(January):357.
2. Lazarou J, Pomeranz BH, Corey PN. Incidence of adverse drug reactions in hospitalized patients: A meta-analysis of prospective studies. *JAMA.* 1998;5(279):1200-1205.
3. Centers for Disease Control, National Center for Health Statistics http://www.cdc.gov/nchs/fastats/lcod.htm
4. American Heart Association: http://www.americanheart.org/
5. American Cancer Society: http://www.cancer.org/
6. Starfield, B. Is U.S. health really the best in the world? *JAMA.* 2000;284(4):483-485
7. Buser H, Muller MD, Theobald N. Occurrence of the pharmaceutical drug Clofibric acid and the herbicide Mecoprop in various Swiss lakes and in the North Sea. *Environ Sci Technol* 1998;31(1):188-192.
8. Raloff J. Drugged waters–does it matter that pharmaceuticals are turning up in water supplies? *Science News.* March 21, 1998, Volume 153.
9. Ternes T. Pharmaceutical residues in the environment–much ado about nothing? Institute for Water Research & Technology 1998: www.epa.gov/nerlesd1/chemistry/ppcp/ images/ternes-security.pdf
10. Hartman A. Identification of fluoroquinolone antibiotics as the main source of umuC genotoxicity in native hospitals. *Environ Toxicol Chem* 1998;17(3):377-382.
11. Nicolopoulou P, Pitsos MA. The impact of endocrine disruptors in the human reproductive system. Hum Reprod Update 2001;7(3):323-330.
12. Snyder S. Toxicant identification and evaluation (TIE) of endocrine disrupters in aqueous mixtures. *Soc Environ Toxicol Chem.* November, 1997.
13. Thompson D. Killer Bacteria. *Time* magazine. August 3, 1998:152(5).
14. Spake A. Losing the battle of the bugs. *U.S. News and World Report,* May 10, 1999.
15. Ott WR, Roberts, JW. Everyday exposure to toxic pollutants. *Scientific American;* Feb 1998:86-91.

Additional reading:
Webb Nicholas J. *The Cost of Being Sick.* Sounds Concepts. Orem, Utah 2003.

Chapter 8
Can You Eat 100 Pounds of Liver a Day?

We have clearly established the relationship between certain stress factors, especially environmental stress and diseases. Now let's look at disease statistics from around the world before we get to "The Solution" section of this book. I want to be absolutely sure that every reader of this book understands how serious this threat is, and that diet alone can no longer provide more than a fraction of what we need to maintain health, let alone fight disease. There are many actions we must take for our individual health as well as for the health of this planet.

Around the world, oxidative stress is the principal cause of degenerative diseases like cancers and heart disease. There is an increasing body of evidence that oxidative stress may also be contributing to other problems like cognitive dysfunction (such as ADHD and ADD), diabetes and other diseases and conditions that are worsening worldwide. You have read a great deal about what's happening in North America. What follows is some information about other nations that I have visited, as well as some data gathered from their health agencies.

Cancer is a Major Burden on Australia.
Cancer in Australia from 1990 to 2000:
- Cancer has risen in Australian women by 30%.
- Cancer has risen in Australian men by 33%.
- 29% of men and 25% of women die of cancer.
- One in every three Australian men is affected by cancer during the first 75 years of life.
- One in every four Australian women is affected by cancer during the first 75 years of life.

  – Australian Institute of Health and Welfare, 2000[1]

New Zealand, Do You Think You are Well?
- 16% have asthma.
- 60% see their doctors two to five times a year.
- 69% take at least one prescription drug.

  – New Zealand Statistics[2]

Heart Disease is a Major Burden on New Zealand.
- 43% of New Zealanders die of heart disease.
- 48% of males and 36% of females have excess central obesity.

  – New Zealand Health Information Service, 1998[3]

Cancer in New Zealand from 1997 to 1998
- 8,842 new cancer cases in New Zealand women.
- 7,689 new cancer cases in New Zealand men.
- 27% of New Zealanders die of cancer.

  – New Zealand Health Information Service, 1998[3]

Heart Disease in the United Kingdom
- Heart and circulatory disease is the UK's biggest killer.
- 40% of deaths in the UK are from heart disease.
  - British Heart Foundation, 2004[4]

Cancer in the UK
- 26% of all deaths in the UK are from cancer.
- In 2002, there were 155,180 deaths from cancer in the UK.
- 31% of men in the UK under the age of 65 die from cancer.
- 47% of women in the UK under the age of 65 die from cancer.
  - Cancer Research UK, 2003[5]

Cancer Statistics–Canada
- On average, 2,690 Canadians are diagnosed with cancer every week.
- On average, 1,296 Canadians die of cancer every week.
- Since 1988, breast cancer incidence rates have risen by 10%.
  - Canadian Cancer Society, 2003[6]

Cancer in the United States
- 24% of all deaths in the U.S. are from cancer.
- Over 18 million new cases of cancer have been diagnosed since 1990.
- In 2004, more than 1,500 people a day will die of cancer.
  - U.S. Centers for Disease Control, 2004[7]

Cancer: Risk Factors
- Smoking–approximately one-third of cancer deaths.
- Diet–approximately one-quarter of cancer deaths.
- Up to 10% of cancer deaths can be traced to genetics.
  - The National Cancer Institute (NCI), 2004[8]

These facts from NCI total only 68%. What are the other risks? In my opinion, based on the data you are reading in this book, it is the toxins present in our air, water and food.

21st-Century America
- One out of every two people will get heart disease.
- One out of every three Americans will get cancer.
- 50 million Americans have autoimmune disease.
- All degenerative diseases are on the rise.
  - U.S. CDC, NCI, DHHS, 2004[7,8,9]

Breast Cancer in the United States
Over 300,000 American women are diagnosed with breast cancer each year. Breast cancer takes between 5 and 30 years of growth in the body before it can be diagnosed as a cancer.
  - The National Cancer Institute, 2004[8]

As mentioned earlier, one out of every three Americans will get cancer. This is a certainty. But the statistics are similar in other modern nations, as well. If you look at the figures just listed, you will see that the numbers for Canada, Australia and New Zealand are also quite frightening.

According to government statistics from the United Kingdom, one in every three people will develop cancer in the UK, and 26% of the population will die from cancer.

Smoking is believed to cause approximately one-third of cancer deaths in the U.S. Approximately one-quarter of total cancer deaths can be attributed to diet. The remaining cancers can be attributed to infection, chemicals and pollutants.[10]

Breast cancer in the United States is serious, but in the United Kingdom it's almost unbelievable. The mortality rate for breast cancer in the UK is the highest in Western Europe. England and Wales have the highest rates of breast cancer in the entire world. And the death rate from breast cancer there is currently increasing by .5% per year.[11]

Lung cancer in Scotland is much higher than it is in England and Wales: Scotland, 97.2 per 100,000 males; Northern England, 79.0 per 100,000 males; Southwest England, 42.3 per 100,000 males. Male mortality is twice as high as female mortality, but it is declining, whereas female mortality from lung cancer in Scotland and England is increasing. Mortality in the UK from lung cancer is 40% higher than elsewhere in Europe.[11]

Heart disease is also a free radical, oxidative stress disease. According to the World Cancer Research Fund, 300,000 people die from heart disease and cancer in the United Kingdom each year. That group says that just one serving per day of whole grains could cut deaths by 24,000 per year.[12]

As governments search for answers, there has been enough research progress to identify that diet is a significant factor in free radical degenerative disease. However, most researchers are not yet aware that it is impossible to eat enough food to get sufficient antioxidants to protect our bodies from the toxic threat that exists on our planet today. Since antioxidants can render disease-causing free radicals from toxins harmless, they are crucial to our health.

Dr. Les Packer, a world-renowned expert in antioxidant research, states that it is virtually impossible to eat enough food to receive sufficient antioxidants to protect us from the ravages of free radical disease, such as cancer and heart disease, in today's environment.[13] He then offers a couple of examples. One is vitamin E, a commonly accepted and scientifically validated antioxidant nutrient.

Dr. Packer explains that you would have to eat about 100 pounds of liver per day, or 125 tablespoons of peanut butter oil per day, to get sufficient vitamin E for even minimal protection. Or you could take a dietary supplement. *(Hmmm...Is that a tough choice?)*

He also states that, in conjunction with glutathione (another important antioxidant discussed in more detail later in this book), it is impossible to eat enough food to get sufficient glutathione protection each day. This idea will be revisited again in "The Solution" section of this book.

We are seeing trends in degenerative disease that no one could ever have imagined before the age of synthetic chemistry.

Internationally famous TV journalist Bill Moyers, who now works for PBS, has produced some excellent work to alert America to our environmental problems, beginning with a series of programs called "Trade Secrets."[14] In these programs, Mr. Moyers did an excellent job exposing the strong link between various chemical toxins and many diseases and illnesses. At the end of one program, he allowed himself to be tested. A serum analysis was done, testing for a total of 150 possible toxins. Eighty-four toxins were found in his blood.

The doctor who performed the test said that if they had tested for additional toxins, they would have undoubtedly found more. Of course, Mr. Moyers has not spent his life in factories or working near toxic waste sites. Although he has been a reporter in the field, he has had no more extraordinary exposure to chemicals than the average person and certainly less than factory workers. Yet at least 84 toxins were found in his blood stream.

I strongly recommend Mr. Moyers' work on toxins. You can obtain transcripts from PBS, or better yet, you can purchase these programs on videotape from PBS. I urge you to get these programs and watch them so that you can understand how serious the threat to your health and to the health of your children really is.

It doesn't matter where you live, you can't escape toxins. As we established earlier, our home is no longer the safest place to be.

Free radicals are produced normally as a by-product of energy production. But chemicals in the environment are causing free radical activity far over and above the limits that our bodies were designed to handle. One expert in oxidative stress, Dr. Bruce Ames, says that the human body is now taking approximately 10,000 free radical hits to its DNA and every cell in the body every day.[15]

We take toxic chemicals into our body in incredibly small amounts daily–which, of course, is why government officials tell us not to worry. It takes many years for these toxins to accumulate to the point where they can either suppress the immune system or cause immune system dysfunction. Eventually our bodies may fall victim to some opportunistic mechanism, such as cancer, mutated viruses or medication-resistant bacteria.

The EPA releases air pollutant statistics and other sources of pollution by state. I will refer to some maps and charts in a moment. The toxins in question, found in higher levels in the Western portion of the U.S. at this time, are relatively new to that region. But these toxins have been in the Eastern section of the U.S. since the age of synthetic chemistry began in 1930.10 The first time I made maps of the type you are about to view was in 1987, then updated them in 1997. Looking at those older maps, there was very little cancer concentration comparatively in the West as opposed to the Eastern United States, where the toxins had been present far longer. I used to tell my audiences that, "Eventually, disease statistics will be far higher in the West than in the East simply because of the time of exposure to either suspected or known cancer-causing agents in the air". Keep in mind that the maps and charts we are about to look at do not reflect is only a measurement of all known sources of disease-causing toxins. air-polluting, cancer-causing agents. This doesn't even address the amount of cancer-causing agents currently found in drinking water or the agents are found in your home due to various factors previously mentioned. Nor does it address the . In addition, cancer-causing agents that are known to exist in many some foods.

Please refer to the series of maps (Plates 7 through 11) at the center of the book. The first map shows the death rate from all forms of cancer in the continental US per hundred thousand people (per capita) by county, the deeper the red the higher the deaths per capita. The next map, Plate 8, shows (again by county) toxins (in green) known to be linked to cancer. The overlap is alarming and the correlation is obvious. The next map shows breast cancer by county in white females. Yes other get breast cancer including small percentages of makes of all races, but unfortunately at the time of printing I did have the time or resources to do this for the world in all races and genders. These should help to make the point for now however.

Plates 7 through 9 deal with toxins of all types that cause or contribute to cancers from all sources, including air, water, food, building materials, etc. The next two maps, plates 10 and 11, deal with toxins emitted in the air only. Plate 10 shows the emission of all known air pollutants that threaten human life from all diseases and disorders. These include air pollutants that are known or suspected to cause cancer as well as those that affect the nervous system and the immune system in general, which as a result my contribute to virtually any health challenge, from chronic fatigue to cancer. Plate 10 also includes those toxin emissions that are known or suspected to contribute to behavioral and learning problems in adults as well as children, such as ADD and ADHD. Many of these toxins are also known or suspected to be endocrine disruptors, feminizing chemicals that can affect fertility in males, and lastly those chemicals known to cause or contribute to respiratory diseases, such as asthma and allergies.

Plate 11 concentrates on toxic air emissions that affect the respiratory tract only, denoted by state. I will refer again to the maps labeled Plate 10 and Plate 11 later when we discuss air pollution and air quality issues in chapter 12.

After more than a quarter of a century as a health educator, I have realized that some people learn better with pictures (hence the maps), and some do better with statistical charts and/or graphs. So the next thing you'll be looking at is the latest data reported by state (as of the time of this printing) for toxin release that affect or cause the following:

- Cancers of all types
- Dioxin releases
- Toxins suspected to cause neurological disorders
- Toxins that cause reproductive disorders (infertility and endocrine disruption)
- Toxins that are suspected (some known) to cause respiratory disorders

Most everyone wants to know just where their home state ranks in terms of air quality, and most everyone is surprised to find out where they rank. Why? As I have mentioned and will continue to repeat, the majority of toxins that adversely affect your health and even cause disease are chemicals you cannot see and often cannot taste or smell. Out of sight/out of mind, as the saying goes. And once again the level of awareness about how toxins affect your health is almost nil in government (except of course for the EPA) in the healthcare community, the media and therefore the general public. EPA is doing the best they can with what they have to work with, but let's face it: How many citizens visit the EPA Web site daily for updates? Most government officials outside of EPA either don't know the problem exists, or they are tasked with telling the public that it isn't really a problem. Unfortunately most environmentalists have been so radical and one-sided in their efforts that the word environmentalist conjures up only negative responses at all levels. These negative reactions range from jokes about "environmental whackos" to a defensive posture to protect world capitalism from assault by perceived anarchists.

It is the case with every movement that subjective extremists are present, but even they have accomplished some good in getting many issues brought to where they are today. I am endeavoring to get those who have previously had knee-jerk, negative reactions to environmentalists to read this information and simply begin to do their parts to ensure both personal and world health.

U.S. PIRG (Public Interest Research Groups) Toxic Report Releases and Health: A Review of Pollution Data and Current Knowledge on the Health Effects of Toxic Chemicals, January 22, 2003 U.S. PIRG Education Fund.

Figure 1
Cancer-Causing Chemical Releases in 2000 by State (pounds)

State	Air	Water	Total	Rank
TX	8,644,611	69,057	8,713,668	1
PA	6,232,498	43,262	6,275,761	2
IN	6,214,965	50,150	6,265,116	3
OH	5,778,617	58,989	5,837,606	4
TN	4,935,687	99,043	5,034,730	5
MS	4,901,334	22,077	4,923,411	6
SC	4,221,542	101,150	4,322,692	7
NC	4,191,609	102,167	4,293,776	8
LA	4,162,329	87,161	4,249,490	9
FL	4,162,021	33,670	4,195,690	10
IL	3,904,543	13,923	3,918,466	11
GA	3,259,232	65,823	3,325,055	12
AL	3,122,108	121,474	3,243,582	13
VA	3,086,556	28,859	3,115,415	14
KY	2,479,622	109,236	2,588,859	15
PR	2,507,428	9,084	2,516,633	16
NY	2,202,428	156,361	2,358,789	17
OR	2,275,604	10,470	2,286,074	18
WI	2,163,656	21,667	2,185,323	19
CA	2,025,868	82,225	2,108,093	20
MO	1,873,458	20,144	1,893,602	21
MI	1,747,061	20,697	1,767,758	22
WA	1,627,993	94,558	1,722,551	23
CT	1,407,135	6,565	1,413,701	24
AR	1,225,154	49,708	1,274,862	25
NJ	1,101,762	48,508	1,150,270	26
WV	1,039,441	110,478	1,149,920	27
KS	1,072,749	1,884	1,074,633	28
OK	927,285	2,923	930,209	29
IA	884,978	21,567	906,545	30
MN	888,773	12,248	901,021	31
MT	740,649	770	741,418	32
MD	628,605	22,293	650,898	33
ME	560,063	21,154	581,217	34
MA	514,781	61,368	576,149	35
UT	301,404	4,992	306,397	36
DE	295,281	4,633	299,915	37
AZ	189,629	531	189,705	38
NH	183,629	3,444	187,073	39
NE	147,890	1,510	149,400	40
RI	112,666	341	113,006	41
NV	107,078	5,277	112,355	42
ID	86,343	12,084	98,427	43
ND	70,101	23,156	93,257	44
HI	87,368	64	87,432	45
CO	80,737	819	81,557	46
NM	65,958	337	66,295	47
WY	56,979	466	57,445	48
AK	40,225	594	40,819	49
VI	32,540	3	32,543	50
SD	17,450	801	18,251	51
GU	3,913	0	3,913	52
VT	1,493	0	1,502	53
MP	1,240	0	1,240	54
DC	8	0	8	55

Figure 2
Dioxin Releases in 2000 by State (grams)

State	Air	Water	Total	Rank
TX	528.5	602.3	1,130.8	1
LA	103.5	934.7	1,038.2	2
AL	902.3	130.7	1,032.9	3
GA	994.6	19.6	1,104.2	4
UT	658.4	0.0	658.4	5
NE	432.2	0.0	432.2	6
MS	20.4	176.2	196.6	7
IN	190.7	0.0	190.8	8
PA	173.2	4.5	177.7	9
VA	104.3	6.7	111.0	10
SC	98.4	5.7	104.0	11
WA	40.3	44.3	84.6	12
FL	70.6	4.4	75.0	13
NC	69.0	3.5	72.4	14
WV	66.6	2.8	69.4	15
OK	67.9	0.2	68.1	16
TN	49.6	16.1	65.7	17
WI	62.0	0.8	62.8	18
OH	53.4	2.78	56.2	19
IA	51.0	0.0	51.0	20
MD	34.1	16.3	50.4	21
IL	50.0	0.0	50.0	22
KS	46.1	0.7	46.8	23
AR	29.1	12.1	41.2	24
KY	35.2	5.1	40.3	25
NY	32.6	6.3	38.9	26
CA	34.6	4.1	38.7	27
OR	8.8	24.6	33.3	28
MI	25.2	5.8	31.1	29
MO	27.2	2.9	30.2	30
DE	5.0	14.0	19.0	31
PR	16.5	0.0	16.5	32
MT	16.1	0.2	16.3	33
WY	15.2	0.0	15.2	34
ME	8.7	6.2	14.9	35
AZ	14.2	0.0	14.2	36
SD	1.1	12.6	13.7	37
MA	11.7	0.1	11.7	38
NV	10.9	0.0	10.9	39
CT	7.6	3.0	10.6	40
NJ	8.0	0.5	8.6	41
MN	8.3	0.0	8.3	42
CO	8.3	0.1	8.3	43
NM	8.0	0.0	8.0	4.4
ND	7.7	0.0	7.7	45
ID	1.9	5.1	7.0	46
HI	4.9	0.0	4.9	47
NH	1.4	0.7	2.1	48
VT	1.1	0.0	1.1	49
VI	1.0	0.1	1.1	50
AK	0.5	0.0	0.5	51
DC	0.1	0.0	0.1	52
RI	0.0	0.0	0.0	53

U.S. PIRG (Public Interest Research Groups) Toxic Report Releases and Health: A Review of Pollution Data and Current Knowledge on the Health Effects of Toxic Chemicals, January 22, 2003 U.S. PIRG Education Fund.

Figure 3
Suspected Neurological Toxic Releases in 2000 by State (pounds)

State	Air	Water	Total	Rank
TX	84,468,530	1,373,996	85,842,526	1
TN	65,817,360	1,007,192	66,824,552	2
LA	60,398,444	1,555,113	61,953,557	3
OH	55,784,338	876,221	56,660,560	4
AL	45,713,387	1,342,420	47,055,808	5
IN	45,618,603	602,140	46,220,743	6
GA	45,302,599	848,937	46,151,535	7
UT	44,618,462	13,045	44,631,507	8
IL	40,808,804	217,056	41,025,861	9
NC	39,384,934	1,112,336	40,497,270	10
SC	36,354,427	812,973	37,167,399	11
VA	36,009,751	453,560	36,463,311	12
FL	33,063,688	320,614	33,384,302	13
MI	31,718,810	450,592	32,169,402	14
PA	30,449,939	401,136	30,851,075	15
MS	29,025,929	518,363	29,644,292	16
KY	26,533,313	349,999	26,883,312	17
MO	25,501,624	417,054	25,918,678	18
AR	23,175,171	882,166	24,057,336	19
CA	20,403,394	2,145,839	22,549,233	20
WI	19,911,101	293,232	20,204,333	21
IA	18,812,556	399,056	19,211,612	22
OK	17,040,928	140,013	17,180,941	23
WA	15,577,240	1,037,113	16,614,535	24
OR	15,751,540	191,101	15,942,641	25
KS	14,640,883	115,038	14,755,921	26
WV	12,877,644	1,206,421	14,084,064	27
NY	13,559,157	494,293	14,053,450	28
MN	13,136,134	232,186	13,368,320	29
NJ	9,745,876	472,832	10,218,708	30
MD	7,738,537	487,961	8,226,498	31
PR	7,969,851	6,915	7,976,766	32
NE	5,654,542	218,857	5,873,399	33
ME	5,071,827	418,533	5,490,360	34
MT	5,145,185	46,466	5,191,650	35
ID	4,992,830	163,727	5,156,557	36
MA	4,037,791	99,493	4,137,283	37
CT	3,633,571	40,483	3,674,054	38
AZ	3,043,629	5,351	3,048,980	39
CO	2,731,928	46,320	2,778,248	40
ND	2,473,726	49,850	2,523,576	41
AK	2,435,819	67,481	2,503,30	42
NH	2,316,348	95,038	2,411,386	43
DE	2,330,439	65,682	2,396,121	44
SD	1,956,317	6,783	1,963,100	45
NV	1,936,881	22,107	1,958,988	46
WY	1,416,988	16,049	1,433,037	47
RI	926,538	755	927,293	48
NM	730,514	699	731,213	49
VI	508,830	38,403	547,233	50
HI	269,742	1,204	270,946	51
VT	116,682	7,867	124,549	52
GU	19,087	0	19,087	53
AS	16,780	0	16,780	54
MP	7,990	0	7,990	55
DC	8	74	82	56

Figure 4
Reproductive Toxic Releases in 2000 by State (pounds)

State	Air	Water	Total	Rank
TN	20,069,429	9,052	20,078,481	1
AL	11,588,394	4,532	11,592,926	2
IL	3,873,457	3,002	3,876,459	3
TX	2,977,191	6,823	2,984,014	4
KS	1,565,398	828	1,566,226	5
AR	1,414,650	7,999	1,422,649	6
LA	1,210,565	3,801	1,214,366	7
WV	832,455	3,901	836,356	8
NY	819,735	3,638	823,373	9
OH	686,001	8,242	694,243	10
GA	562,845	1,199	564,044	11
MO	533,282	6,945	540,227	12
PA	463,497	13,463	476,960	13
FL	469,594	978	470,572	14
WI	464,212	909	465,121	15
SC	432,339	19,778	452,117	16
IN	314,311	7,190	321,501	17
NJ	303,106	1,658	304,764	18
MI	292,117	632	292,749	19
VA	241,630	10,663	252,293	20
KY	220,942	9,557	230,499	21
UT	119,403	1,488	120,891	22
WA	119,066	700	119,766	23
OK	115,794	605	116,399	24
CA	89,246	1,235	90,481	25
MS	85,385	483	85,868	26
PR	80,575	16	80,591	27
ND	41,406	17,337	58,743	28
NC	49,975	6,871	56,846	29
AZ	52,150	16	52,166	30
MN	49,626	67	49,693	31
NM	43,470	3	43,473	32
NV	41,086	60	41,146	34
MT	41,053	11	41,064	34
WY	40,212	262	40,474	35
AK	38,400	435	38,835	36
VI	36,097	1	36,098	37
IA	31,977	220	32,197	38
NH	31,393	262	31,655	39
MA	29,409	314	29,723	40
DE	28,193	162	28,355	41
HI	27,411	20	27,431	42
CT	25,640	328	25,968	43
MD	21,305	4,082	25,387	44
OR	21,826	935	22,761	45
CO	17,643	103	17,746	46
NE	14,560	105	14,665	47
ID	8,836	839	9,675	48
RI	8,469	12	8,481	49
ME	6,093	18	6,111	50
GU	3,440	0	3,440	51
MP	1,240	0	1,240	52
SD	1,104	5	1,109	53
VT	5	9	14	54

U.S. PIRG (Public Interest Research Groups) Toxic Report Releases and Health: A Review of Pollution Data and Current Knowledge on the Health Effects of Toxic Chemicals, January 22, 2003 U.S. PIRG Education Fund.

Figure 5
Suspected Respiratory Toxic Releases in 2000 by State (pounds)

State	Air Emission	Rank
OH	133,325,669	1
NC	124,650,411	2
GA	94,612,247	3
PA	92,996,650	4
FL	86,318,614	5
IN	85,218,750	6
TX	82,916,656	7
TN	80,682,391	8
WV	71,799,135	9
MI	68,359,686	10
AL	67,878,236	11
KY	66,327,729	12
LA	63,850,151	13
IL	60,512,782	14
VA	57,126,815	15
SC	53,744,745	16
UT	48,912,957	17
MS	42,551,517	18
MO	35,903,445	19
MD	33,860,843	20
NY	31,470,735	21
WI	28,319,232	22
AR	23,887,688	23
CA	21,723,478	24
IA	21,522,805	25
OK	18,363,490	26
WA	17,442,906	27
PR	17,237,508	28
NJ	15,904,089	29
OR	15,832,450	30
KS	14,882,875	31
MN	14,148,060	32
MA	9,079,875	33
NE	7,792,084	34
DE	7,242,927	35
ME	6,322,936	36
MT	6,050,295	37
NH	5,376,767	38
ID	5,270,149	39
AZ	4,904,689	40
CT	4,736,345	41
CO	3,613,635	42
ND	3,145,916	43
NV	2,958,964	44
AK	2,692,469	45
SD	2,027,682	46
WY	1,907,549	47
NM	1,159,072	48
HI	1,022,580	49
RI	944,788	50
VI	460,180	51
GU	223,797	52
VT	117,713	53
DC	53,008	54
AS	16,780	55
MP	7,990	56

Figure 6
Developmental Toxic Releases in 2000 by State (pounds)

State	Air	Water	Total	Rank
TN	27,926,717	21,448	27,948,165	1
AL	13,678,522	49,641	13,728,163	2
IL	8,095,783	3,842	8,099,625	3
TX	7,493,649	32,506	7,526,155	4
IN	6,484,257	19,762	6,504,019	5
NC	4,923,452	20,550	4,944,002	6
SC	4,634,688	30,741	4,665,429	7
PA	4,542,023	10,182	4,552,206	8
VA	4,455,462	21,358	4,476,820	9
MI	3,993,947	3,823	3,997,770	10
KY	3,831,755	47,303	3,879,058	11
LA	3,653,721	9,280	3,663,001	12
OH	3,626,791	20,757	3,647,548	13
MS	3,588,857	1,337	3,590,194	14
NY	3,138,210	10,906	3,149,116	15
AR	2,985,826	8,403	2,994,228	16
GA	2,932,112	6,677	2,938,788	17
WI	2,806,119	1,563	2,807,682	18
KS	2,773,414	950	2,774,364	19
FL	2,410,250	1,880	2,412,130	20
MO	2,347,132	8,150	2,355,282	21
NJ	2,011,500	31,712	2,043,212	22
WV	1,773,792	8,523	1,782,314	23
OK	1,703,977	904	1,704,881	24
IA	1,698,113	2,297	1,700,410	25
MN	1,689,479	75	1,689,554	26
MA	1,143,186	687	1,143,873	27
CA	953,797	1,683	955,480	28
CT	857,722	330	858,052	29
WA	754,340	1,126	755,466	30
PR	599,390	48	539,438	31
NE	472,533	105	472,638	32
NV	450,478	3,856	454,334	33
OR	401,012	1,771	402,783	34
UT	294,791	1,747	296,538	35
ID	283,198	1,152	284,350	36
MD	277,128	5,267	282,395	37
ME	265,417	49	265,466	38
CO	247,446	125	247,571	39
NH	198,372	276	198,648	40
RI	182,875	32	182,907	41
NM	181,460	4	181,464	42
AZ	153,316	17	153,133	43
SD	146,415	574	146,989	44
ND	116,689	20,965	137,654	45
WY	108,180	522	108,702	46
MT	89,981	50	90,030	47
VI	78,958	1	78,959	48
DE	72,112	230	73,341	49
AK	64,392	698	65,090	50
HI	60,122	44	60,166	51
VT	21,028	229	21,257	52
GU	9,006	0	9,006	53
MP	3,986	0	3,986	54
DC	8	0	8	55

U.S. PIRG (Public Interest Research Groups) Toxic Report Releases and Health: A Review of Pollution Data and Current Knowledge on the Health Effects of Toxic Chemicals, January 22, 2003 U.S. PIRG Education Fund.

Figure 7
Carcinogen Releases in 2000
by Industry Sector (pounds)

Industry	Air	Water	Total
Plastics Foam Products	18,942,129	5	18,942,134
Industrial Organic Chemicals, NEC	7,094,810	156,469	7,251,278
Pulp Mills	6,396,524	343,878	6,740,402
Reconstituted Wood, Products	5,552,142	1,101	5,553,243
Plastics Materials and Resins	4,529,880	108,735	4,638,615
Paper Mills	3,902,474	198,116	4,100,589
Paperboard Mills	3,763,525	45,556	3,809,081
Petroleum Refining	3,106,385	42,103	3,202,488
Pharmaceutical Preparations	2,851,794	1,950	2,853,745
Electric Services	1,731,458	481,611	2,213,068

Figure 8
Dioxin Releases in 2000
by Industry Sector (grams)

Industry	Air	Water	Total
Alkalies Chlorine	162	1,422	1,583
Secondary Nonferrous Metals	1,098	0	1,098
Organic Fibers, Noncellulosic	808	0	808
Electric Services	677	0	677
Primary Nonferrous Metals, NEC	624	0	624
Electric and Other services Combined	470	0	470
Cement, Hydraulic	447	1	448
Wood Preserving	12	357	369
Industrial Organic Chemicals, NEC	186	87	272
Pulp Mills	60	115	175

Figure 9
Suspected Neurological Toxin Releases
in 2000 by Industry Sector (pounds)

Industry	Air	Water	Total
Pulp Mills	75,256,626	6,812,285	82,068,912
Electric Services	65,199,476	965,827	6,616,503
Industrial Organic Chemicals, NEC	50,817,506	1,600,853	52,418,359
Primary Nonferrous Metals, NEC	47,210,612	167,685	47,378,297
Paperboard Mills	44,932,457	1,299,062	46,231,519
Nitrogenous Fertilizers	42,871,641	554,015	43,425,656
Petroleum Refining	38,837,160	1,067,728	39,904,888
Paper Mills	35,252,953	2,160,067	37,413,020
Motor Vehicles and Car Bodies	32,390,187	1,798	32,391,985
Cellulosic Manmade Fibers	31,269,004	250,383	31,519,387

Figure 10
Suspected Respiratory Toxin Releases
in 2000 by Industry Sector (pounds)

Industry	Air Emissions
Electric Services	115,948,940
Pulp Mills	87,076,027
Paperboard Mills	51,247,786
Primary Nonferrous Metals, NEC	49,308,665
Industrial Organic Chemicals, NEC	46,648,437
Paper Mills	46,111,887
Petroleum Refining	44,310,309
Nitrogenous Fertilizers	43,631,655
Motor Vehicles and Car Bodies	36,010,314
Plastic Materials and Resins	26,852,371

We need everyone from all points of view to realize that life on planet Earth is literally at stake. We are running out of time and must all work together, or we will all fail together. I have included information in this book's Solution section on all the many hopeful things we can all do. I have included health, economic and environmental motivations. I don't care who you are, what political party you belong to, or what your personal views. We need to unite or this beautiful blue planet will become a massive orbiting graveyard around our sun—and this tragedy is likely to happen within this 21st century if we don't all start working together without delay. Ignoring these issues will not make them go away, and you cannot hope that a small handful of concerned people will solve the problem for the rest of the world. If there was ever a reason for human beings to see themselves **not** as individuals or particular nationalities, ethnic groups or religions, *this is it!*

Remember in chapter 5 I gave an example of just how little it takes to affect our health, and that we cannot in most cases detect those levels with our senses. It is worth repeating that example here. Most people can start to smell benzene in the air at 1.5–4.7 parts of benzene per million parts of air (ppm). They can smell benzene in water at 2 ppm. The EPA has set the maximum permissible level of benzene in drinking water at 5 parts per billion (ppb). One ppb is one 1000th of a ppm. Therefore, long before you can smell benzene, you will have already far exceeded safe levels. Most people can't begin to taste benzene in water until it reaches 0.5–4.5 ppm–again, far beyond safe levels.

When we add items that may contribute to immune or nervous system dysfunction, correlation with the highest rates of death per capita becomes much stronger. This fact presents a very persuasive case that toxins in the environment can affect your health.

Before I go any further, I want to reinforce the fact that although toxins are obviously the single most serious threat to life on this planet today, they are not the sole factor. As I have stated throughout this book, there are multiple factors contributing to the whole. These factors range from nutritional deficiencies to lifestyle choices, as well as home and work environments.

For some people, genes also play a role. Many cancers in adults under age 40 have a significant inherited factor. Up to one in every 10 cases of cancer of the ovary, breast, prostate and colorectal system is due in part to the inheritance of abnormal genes. The toxins then act simply as triggers. Also, the older we get, the greater our risk since the combination of several factors eventually leads to cancer. The most common factors are total exposure and bioaccumulation of carcinogens (cancer-causing agents) over time, such as certain chemicals (particularly those found in tobacco smoke), dietary factors, some viruses and specific types of radiation, including the ultraviolet light in natural sunlight.[8]

In adults over age 50, the total number of newly diagnosed cancer cases roughly doubles each decade. Therefore, an 80-year-old person is eight times more likely to have cancer than someone who is 50 years old.[16] Since the majority of the population is now over 50, this fact will undoubtedly affect the statistics and may be a contributing factor to the estimate that total cancers will rise by as much as 70 percent by the year 2010.

Take Responsibility for Your Own Health

Clearly this is the time when we must do everything we can to protect ourselves and to be proactive about maintaining our health. **That means more than just diet and exercise. In today's world, we must have dietary supplements–supplements that are scientifically validated to give us the support we need.**

Sadly, there are individuals who always want to leave the responsibility for their lives and health in someone else's hands. Perhaps they are too lazy or just not interested. It's difficult to say why people make the decisions they make. Perhaps they tell themselves, "Well, I feel fine, I'll deal with it tomorrow." Or, "It's okay if I eat this bad food today. I'll make up for it next week." Or, "I don't believe it will threaten my health if I smoke cigarettes, or eat food that has known toxins in it." The one that really tickles me is, "I'm not worried. The government will protect me."

Industry creates billions of tons of highly toxic (including some deadly) waste annually. Since there is only so much land mass, how do they dispose of this dangerous stuff? One of the most common practices is to mix toxins into farm fertilizer. Now, of course, the "experts" say that the amount of radioactive waste and other toxins put into the farm fertilizer is so minuscule that it couldn't possibly hurt you. They tell us, "The average human can absorb and tolerate it without any problem, so it's not a danger." In fact, according to these same experts, this is a very positive and productive way to get rid of nuclear waste and heavy metals.

I know of several states where at least 18 known toxic metals and various types of industrial wastes, as well as radioactive waste material, are being mixed into farm fertilizers and sold to unsuspecting farmers. No, there are no label warnings or disclosures required by law.

I must emphasize that not every farm uses the same brands of fertilizer, and therefore not every farm in each of those states uses toxic fertilizer on their crops. The fact that this occurs at all is a wake-up call for everyone–consumers and farmers alike (Plate 12).

A courageous article was printed in *The Seattle Times* on the 4th of July 1997.[17] This article was written by a reporter named Duff Wilson, who described the practice of creating and using toxic fertilizer in detail. This article is still archived on the newspaper's Web site. (at least it still was at the time of this printing). Mr. Wilson deserves kudos for his courageous and excellent work, and I am including some of that information in this section.

Highly toxic steel mill waste, which is approximately 3.6% lead on average, is routinely disposed of nationwide on our farms.[17] Those who defend the practice of using toxic fertilizer say that plants would die from too much zinc before they could absorb the lead, and steel mill waste is approximately 10% zinc on average. Are they right? I don't know, but it makes me very uncomfortable because lead is one of the worst toxins that occurs naturally, and there is already far too much lead in our environment.

As mentioned elsewhere in this book, it is estimated that at least 900,000 American children currently suffer from the toxic effects of lead. Steel mill waste also contains high levels of cadmium. In this book, you have learned that zinc competes with iron and cooper in your blood. Although at first you might say, "Oh good! Extra zinc in my food!" understand that too much zinc can cause very serious, possibly life-threatening, health problems.

Let's look at what can happen:

Radioactive waste from uranium processing has been routinely sprayed on 9,000 acres of grazing land in Gore, Oklahoma. The nuclear power plant fuel processing facility has been closed, but they still spray about 10,000 gallons drawn from the waste pond on grazing land every year. This fertilizer is registered with the State of Oklahoma and contains not only radioactive waste but also 18 toxic heavy metals.[17]

Approximately 400 cows graze on this land, and local residents have linked the bizarre mutations of multi-legged frogs, cows with two noses and more than 120 cases of cancer and birth defects to this state-approved waste disposal practice. State officials and, of course, the company involved say there is no irrefutable proof, and they are correct. As yet there is not conclusive evidence–only correlation exists. But it is an interesting coincidence to say the least.

In Washington state, some of this toxic waste fertilizer was tested on trout by putting a 1% solution in their water. One-hundred percent of the trout died.[17] Of course, trout are much smaller than we are, and we can absorb a lot more toxin before it will kill us.

Cadmium, by the way, is another major health hazard, going into our environment by the billions of tons because of alkaline batteries. This is a problem you can personally help control. When you throw alkaline batteries away, they go into waste disposal sites and break down into the water table. Try using rechargeable batteries that you can recharge thousands of times, and you will help prevent billions of tons of life-threatening waste from entering our world.

How tough would it be to switch? Nearly all of the batteries in my home are rechargeable. I only use alkaline batteries in my smoke detectors. The one-time cost is significant, but your long-term savings in dollars will be far greater. Plus, the life-saving, planet-friendly aspects of this action will be priceless!

Below I've listed states that currently use farm fertilizer that has toxic waste material in it. Depending on the company that makes the fertilizer, it may contain nuclear waste as well as other toxins like cadmium and lead:

- California
- Georgia
- Idaho
- Nebraska
- Oklahoma
- Oregon
- South Carolina
- Washington
- Wyoming

(Once again, please remember that not every farm in these states uses toxic fertilizer.)

The U.S. government has set no limits on how much toxic waste can be put in fertilizer, saying this should be a state-by-state decision.[17]

Scientists desperately seek some other method to dispose of this waste. We can't simply keep burying these waste materials. Fewer and fewer communities are allowing governments and industry to bury toxic waste in their backyards. This is rightly so. Nuclear energy seems to be the favorite solution to energy worldwide. Since governments, including the U.S., seem to think that accumulating nuclear waste is preferable to using fossil fuels, the problem of disposing of nuclear waste won't go away any time soon.

Until we tackle the energy production issue and have the courage to spend the money it will take to convert to truly clean energy, nuclear power plants will continue to spring up around the world like giant radioactive weeds. They contaminate our planet and slowly kill through mutations, birth defects and cancers. No government I know of, including the U.S., wants to face the truth about this fact.

Officials in the U.S. who permit this toxic fertilizer disposal system apparently believe they are doing the right thing. They have convinced themselves that the amounts in the fertilizer are spread thinly by the farmers. The toxins, including radiation, are thin enough that plants, animals and humans can tolerate it. My feeling is that these government officials are generally good people in a bad situation who are seeking the best solution they can find. I am not angry with them, but I am angry with politicians who won't even try to tackle the energy problem. I am also very angry with citizens who abuse energy resources as though they are infinite.

Heavy metals accumulate in your body, as does radioactive material. What many people do not understand is that radioactivity has a given life of the isotope. It will not go away. It will not become neutralized. It will not become safe until its lifespan has expired. It doesn't matter if it goes into farm fertilizer, then into animals, and eventually into us. It doesn't matter how you change the way it's distributed. Radioactivity does not fade away, and it is bioaccumulative in the bodies of all living things.

The toxic waste material put into fertilizer is only a small percentage of the hazards we face. It presents a true problem for the people who need to dispose of it. From their perspective, using it in fertilizer is a safe and reasonable way to dispose of toxic waste. I will make no judgment on this. However, I urge you to think about this fact the next time you go to the polls to vote.

To quote a line from the movie "Indiana Jones and the Last Crusade," "You must choose, but choose wisely".

References
1. Australian Institute of Health and Welfare: http://www.aihw.gov.au/
2. New Zealand Statistics: http://www.stats.govt.nz/domino/external/web/Prod_Serv.nsf/htmldocs/Health
3. New Zealand Health Information Service: http://www.nzhis.govt.nz/
4. British Heart Foundation: http://www.bhf.org.uk/
5. Cancer Research UK: http://www.cancerresearchuk.org/
6. Canadian Cancer Society: http://www.cancer.ca/ccs/
7. U.S. Centers for Disease Control: http://www.cdc.gov/
8. National Cancer Institute: http://www.nci.nih.gov/
9. U.S. Department of Health and Human Services: http://www.hhs.gov/
10. U.S. Environmental Protection Agency: http://www.epa.gov/
11. UK National Statistics Online: http://www.statistics.gov.uk/
12. World Cancer Research Fund: http://www.wcrf-uk.org/
13. Packer L, Colman C. *The Antioxidant Miracle.* John Wiley & Sons, Inc, New York, 1999.
14. Moyers B, Jones S. *Trade Secrets: A Moyers Report.* Public Affairs Television, Inc., 2001: http://pbs.org/tradesecrets/
15. Ames, BN. Endogenous oxidative DNA damage, aging, and cancer. *Free Radic Res Commun* 1989;7:121-128.
16. Goldman DR (ed). *American College of Physicians Complete Home Medical Guide,* 1999. DK Publishing, Inc, New York.
17. Wilson D. Fear in the Fields–How Hazardous Wastes Become Fertilizer–Lack of Fertilizer Regulation in U.S. Leaves Farmers, Consumers Guessing About Toxic Concentrations on Farms. *The Seattle Times*, Business Section, July 1997.

How to Survive on a Toxic Planet

on a

Toxic Planet

SECTION 2

The Solution

Dr. Steve Nugent

Chapter 9
Glyconutritionals–A Sweet Future

This chapter is dedicated to the extremely important subject of glyconutrients. But before I discuss them in detail, I need to clarify some important points about diet and dietary supplements. So please bear with me for a few pages before we get into glyconutrients.

Throughout this book I have emphasized that we live in a place and time when the oxidative stresses we have caused on this planet exceed our bodies' ability to cope unless we provide them with extraordinary assistance.

Our marvelous organic machines were designed to live in an unspoiled world, not on a toxic planet. Our bodies were designed to get the nutrition they need for all functions from fresh, raw natural foods–foods that grew naturally in nutrient-rich soil.

Soil Isn't What It Used To Be
Let's turn to the issue of soil depletion first. Soil depletion is a result of corporate farming methods. For thousands of years, farmers have known that soil rotation was essential to keeping the soil from becoming a useless wasteland. Today, in the name of profits, most corporate farms don't perform required soil maintenance. They simply add three items–nitrogen, phosphorus and potassium (NPK), and sometimes calcium–to the soil. This makes the plants grow full of calories and fiber but void of the complete nutrition you need.

There is unfortunately far too much produce being grown in soil that has less than the full complement of nutrients you need.[1,2] "How can this be?" you might ask. It only takes NPK to make a plant grow, but it takes many more than those three nutrients to make and keep you healthy. Trace minerals are missing or at least deficient in many areas now, and there is little hope of that situation improving in the near future. These trace minerals are required in micrograms, rather than milligrams, but the key word here is "required."

Since heart disease is the number one killer of Americans and number one or two in nearly all modern nations, I'll give you an example of a trace or micromineral important for heart health. Selenium is key to healthy heart function, but most people (and most doctors) are only aware of the importance of vitamin E and the electrolyte minerals (potassium, magnesium, calcium and sodium) for heart health. All the vitamin E in the world is useless without selenium as its partner or synergist.[1,3,4]

Valuable Minerals
Depending on which expert and which source you read, humans need between 42 and 78 different macro- and microminerals each day. All those so-called experts do agree, however, that to be healthy, you must have more than three minerals (NPK) added to our soil and subsequently absorbed by the produce we eat. Minerals are only one category of essential nutrient, but they are often ignored or misunderstood, so they certainly merit further discussion.

Healthy growing plants suck the minerals out of the soil as they grow. Without adequate soil rotation and replenishing methods, that soil will become depleted and lifeless. Quoting U.S. Senate Document #264, published in 1936: "**The alarming fact is that foods (fruits, vegetables and grains) now being raised on millions of acres of land that no longer contain enough of certain minerals are starving us. No matter how much of them we eat, no man today can eat enough fruits and vegetables to sup- ply his system with the minerals he requires for perfect health because his stomach isn't big enough to hold them... The truth is that our foods vary enormously in value, and some of them aren't worth eating as food...**"[5]

The problem of mineral deficiencies in farm soil and therefore plants is increasing around the world. However, few want to recognize this problem. As a result, it is difficult to find all the data you might want on this subject. If you are tenacious enough, you can find some very disturbing information about our soil worldwide and therefore the nutri- tion in the food grown in that soil. Since this book is not specifically dedicated to that, I can only devote a small amount of space to spoil depletion, but I think you probably get the idea.

Commercial farming methods and soil depletion are subjects worthy of their own books, but there are more contributing factors to loss of nutrition than including pro- cessing, cooking, etc., and we will briefly discuss each. In this book I have cited work by Souci, Ramberg and McAnalley on the subject, but right now let's look at work by Bergner. Paul Bergner compiled data from the USDA and other sources to show the decline in mineral and vitamin content of several fruits and vegetables between 1914, 1963, and 1992. Below is a summary of mineral loss from 1963 to 1992 from many dif- ferent causes. He analyzed oranges, apples, bananas, carrots, potatoes, corn, tomatoes, celery, romaine lettuce, broccoli, iceberg lettuce, collard greens and chard.[6]

Average changes in the mineral content of some fruits and vegetables, 1963-1992[6]

Mineral	Average % Change
Calcium	-29.82
Iron	-32.00
Magnesium	-21.08
Phosphorus	-11.09
Potassium	6.48

Our food simply doesn't deliver the nutrition ounce-for-ounce than it did even 40 years ago, and it is a problem that according to scientific documentation continues to get worse every year. It makes one wonder how long it will take before government health officials start recommending dietary supplements daily for everyone.

Unless you farm in the shadow of a volcano or on the nutrient-rich flood plain of a river, it is highly unlikely that the food you grow will provide the nutrition you need. I will discuss this point further in Chapter 10.

To compound the problem, our foods are, in most cases, harvested green so they will have longer shipping and shelf life. However, only fully ripened foods provide the full nutritional potential from the phytochemicals (healthful plant chemicals, not vitamins or minerals) they were designed to yield. This is a critically important fact to know in terms of raw food but less important in terms of dietary supplements. I'll explain what I mean later.

To make the nutrition equation even worse, most people process their food from its natural state, using various methods that involve heat. Such processing reduces nutritional value in proportion to the heat used. This processing includes cooking, canning and drying.[7] If you deplete 90% of the required nutrition from a food through heat, you will have to consume 90% more food to get the minimum required nutrition from it. Who can afford to do that? I don't just mean the cost—I mean who can afford to increase their caloric intake in order to maintain minimum nutrition? Most of the modern world is far too fat already. At the time of printing this book, the U.S. is the fattest nation in the world, with Australia and the UK trailing close behind. No, increasing volume to maintain minimum nutrition is not the answer.

Processing Out Nutrients

Having said that, I know from more than 26 years of lecturing that the above statement, although presented here in writing, will still be misinterpreted. In fact, I have already been misquoted from the first edition of this book, so I'll try explaining this in a different way.

Let's say, for example, that you have only 10% of the lycopene you need from a tomato that was not vine-ripened, was raised in nutrient-poor soil and/or has been heat-treated. This does not mean that you cannot get any lycopene. **It simply means you have to eat ten tomatoes that each contains 10% of the target nutrient rather than one to get the lycopene you need.** The same would be true if you were making a dietary supplement: You would need ten times more raw materials to yield the same amount of lycopene as an optimally healthful tomato.

Companies that do not buy vine-ripened vegetables and fruits, or who treat their raw material with heat or buy from farmers who farm on nutrient-depleted soil, would simply have to buy a much greater volume of raw material. But they could still end up with a target number of milligrams or micrograms of that nutrient in every capsule or tablet. In today's world the quality and potency of a dietary supplement is determined more by quality control measures than by sourcing. Quality control must always be the primary consideration in 21st-century dietary supplements. A professional quality control (QC) department will ensure that the potency and purity you need will be in every serving you consume regardless of the source of the raw materials.

The Quest for Quality

This will no doubt come as a surprise to most consumers, but there are dietary supplement companies that do not have a real quality control department. They may have a QC department on paper, but do they have the equipment and highly trained personnel needed to manage a professional QC function? Almost all companies talk about their quality, but the fact is those statements are based on data at the manufacturer, not from their own QC Department. All companies should have their own (true) QC departments rather than simply relying on the manufacturers' capabilities.

There are thousands of brands of dietary supplements, and only a handful of supplement manufacturers. Most brands you buy are actually identical to hundreds of others.

The only difference is the label. They originate from the same manufacturers and sources. Most of them do not have there own research labs or QC departments–they simply use borrowed data and often even photos of labs at the manufacturer that are not their own. Let the buyer beware!

To emphasize the importance of QC a little further, a group of scientists at the 2001 Nutracon Conference presented data that showed just how poor QC has been in the supplement industry. They randomly purchased major brands and tested only to verify that each product contained the levels of active ingredients listed on each label.

The data that resulted must have shocked even them. They showed as examples:[8]
- *Ephedra* – Zero percent to 154% of label claim.
- *Ginkgo* – Six of 30 products failed.
- *Ginseng* – Tenfold variation to ginsenosides.
- *Yohimbe* – None of the 26 products had an effective level.

It is no small wonder there are so many who believe nutritional support through dietary supplements is merely a phrase. There is, however, very solid science to show that dietary supplementation with the correct nutrients, manufactured with proper QC and administered according to studies rather than randomly, can indeed be extremely effective. I have and will continue to stress that theme with supporting references throughout this book.

Unfortunately in today's world, even organic farms cannot guarantee clean, raw materials since there is no place on the planet that is not exposed to airborne and/or waterborne toxins. Pesticides are in the air, carried on the wind around the globe. Pesticides are nearly always applied by air these days. Unless a farm is in a hermetically sealed dome with the world's most extraordinary air filters bringing in air from outdoors, foods labeled organic will still have pesticides on it. I am not saying so-called organic food is not worth the price. It is simply that it cannot be assumed that, since it was raised with what is inaccurately referred to as organic farming methods, this food is toxin-free. Rather, it means that no toxins have been intentionally applied. That's still very positive and desirable, but it is not a guarantee of being toxin-free. I'll discuss this further shortly.

In the 21st century, all raw materials must be carefully and repeatedly inspected not just for pesticides, but also for toxic metals, synthetic chemicals and microbial organisms. The toxins found must be cleansed from the material if it is to be totally clean. This cleansing, even if done correctly without heat, will still cause a slight loss of nutrition from the raw material. Then the company will have to continually extract whatever active ingredient they need from as much clean, raw material as necessary until they achieve the potency required. That extraction process once again needs to be cold, preferably flash-freezing where possible. Heat is the enemy of nutrition. However, even if heat is used, the goal can still eventually be achieved, but with much more raw material. So, in defense of companies that do not do things the way I would like to see them done, if they have proper quality control, they can still achieve quality target levels.

Let's return to the organic food issue again. Why? Because, as I mentioned earlier, there is no doubt whatsoever in my mind that the above has been misinterpreted by some who think I said organically grown food has no value. Even though I have already covered this issue as it relates to fish farms, there will still be some who believe I have a different meaning than what I explained in that chapter. In any event, one of the most effective ways of learning is through reinforcement by repetition, so this should be both painless and intellectually profitable.

What's Behind the Word "Organic?"

Although we discussed it in Chapter 5, before proceeding let me refresh your memory on the misuse of the word organic. Scientifically speaking, anything that occurs naturally with carbon molecules as part of its molecular structure is organic. All life on this planet is carbon-based, meaning anything that is or ever was alive. So no matter how it was grown, fed or where it came from, all food is technically organic. However, since the common misuse of the term is so widely accepted, I will use the term in this same context, so you will know what I am referring to.

There is a long list of reasons to buy organically raised foods. My wife goes to great pains and expense to do that, so obviously I am in favor of it. Yes, you will pay more, and not just because the sellers know they can charge more. The cost of raising livestock and produce as nature intended in a world that is far from its original design is hugely expensive. (Such a pity…)

I have stated repeatedly and will continue to admonish you that most toxins cannot be seen or detected by human senses at all. Psychologically we want to <u>see</u> the beauty of nature and tell ourselves we are looking at a clean, pure, safe, healthy environment–but that, my friends, is a trap. Later in this book, I will provide examples of how little of a dangerous toxin it takes to attack your health and the levels at which you would see or taste toxins. You will also learn that long before the levels of these toxins are high enough to be detected by human senses, they have already reached dangerous levels in your body. With this fact in mind, as you continue reading please try to suppress the inevitable thought that will go something like, "But my environment looks great, and I feel just fine."

The level of toxin found in organically raised livestock is relatively low considering that all life on this planet, including plant life, is exposed to toxins. Many vegetarians mistakenly believe that by avoiding animal products they will avoid toxins. Many vegetarians quickly get defensive on the issue of their dietary selection, and when people put up psychological defenses they tend not to listen or learn very well. So calm down if you are a vegetarian. I am stating facts and deliberately choosing my words. I mean to say no more or less than what your eyes reveal. Don't read anything into this or make assumptions on what you think I think or think I mean. Okay. Ready?

The fact is that it is very likely that the average human (yes, vegetarians too) already has more toxins in their tissues than the average organically raised cow has. Why? Because we are at the top of the food chain, (remember that concept?) and we outlive most species. Therefore, we have decades to accumulate toxins just a little every day. (Remember those concepts from Chapter 5?)

However, the level of toxins concentrated in <u>commercially</u> raised livestock is frightening when you examine the data. No wonder there are masses of people switching to vegetarianism. They are motivated by that data, and vegetarianism is definitely a valid choice. If their motivation for becoming vegetarian is philosophical or religious, it is simply a choice that I respect and will not argue with. I will not give the full explanation of the true biological design of humans here (as validated by science, not philosophy), since that explanation would no doubt surprise many, and that would digress from the purpose of this book. But I will discuss the subject of human design in great detail in my next book–one that will be dedicated to healthy eating.

It is now possible (for a price) to buy virtually every type of animal and vegetable product you can name grown under organic conditions. In my opinion, it is worth the price in the foods you eat, but not worth the added cost in food supplements.

Is this discussion puzzling you? If you've read many books on nutrition and so-called alternative medicine, you are already accustomed to a subjective, strong, single-minded approach to the topic. Sorry–you won't find that type of approach in anything that I write.

I am an objectivist by nature, not just by training. In case you are unfamiliar with that term, it means I examine all sides of an issue before drawing a conclusion, and that I will make recommendations based on proven facts instead of my personal desires, philosophies or spiritual beliefs (which doesn't always make me happy, I might add). I am not writing this book to push my personal likes, dislikes or philosophies on you and, unlike many popular authors, I am more concerned with being correct than being right.

Am I making my meaning clear? Let's express this thought in another way: I don't need to win. I need you to win. I hope to inform you of facts that you were previously unaware of so that you can make choices that will benefit you, your loved ones and our planet. Yes, you personally can make a difference to our entire planet with your personal choices.

To that end I will attempt to present you with balanced arguments, and if something I say represents my opinion, I will state it as such. I know the objective approach is the worst way to sell books since most people want simple, absolute answers. Although I always endeavor in my lectures and writing to make things as simple and easy to understand as I can, without balance, it simply becomes more rhetoric. Therefore, I do my best to avoid absolutes.

Let's examine the facts: As referenced in this book, the amount of nutrition in foods we eat now is so low as to be of no practical value at all (in most cases) in terms of vitamins, minerals, phytonutrients and glyconutrients. In chapter 10, I discuss this topic in more detail. Today we eat our food for calories and fiber, and even the fiber is lower than it used to be in most foods by weight.[9] **The nutritional value is simply no longer adequate. That is why food supplements are no longer a luxury, but rather a necessity if you wish to have any hope of a long and healthy life as opposed to life support.**

Since toxins are found in the snow of both the north and south poles,[10] there is simply no possibility that any farm anywhere is free of toxin exposure, so all the raw materials should be cleansed regardless of where they came from. And since the nutritional value is so low in produce–even from those labeled organic–the levels of raw material and the extra cost of the organics make the supplement ridiculously expensive. Also, the end-product will be no different, I repeat, no different if the supplement that is made from commercially farmed raw materials goes through the proper steps in quality control for safety, purity and potency. If it is no different, why should you pay more? Let me reinforce here, however, that quality control done properly is in itself expensive, so you need to be a well-educated consumer before you buy.

In regard to the relative safety of the food we eat, organically raised animal products are worth every penny if you consume animal products. This is the case since commercially raised livestock and the products that come from commercial farms and ranches are heavily laden with antibiotics and hormones. The adverse effects of both substances are discussed in several places in this book. Animals raised commercially contain higher amounts of heavy metals and chemicals; in the case of land animals, they are always more fatty. Conversely on average, organically raised animals have as much as 35% less fat by weight, and, in some cases from some farms, even less fat than that. The very significantly lower levels of fat in organically raised land animals is reason enough to change to organically raised meat. Whether you believe that restricting excess fat in your diet helps your weight or heart disease, remember that fat stores toxins that cause disease. **So if you choose to consume animals, always eat lean.**

Go for the Grass-fed Meat

Let's continue for a bit concerning the value of eating organically raised meat as opposed to commercially raised meat. Lower fat, higher EFA content (very important), better flavor, lower probabilities of acid-resistant *E. coli* bacteria transmission, and no difference in tenderness of the meat from the high-fat type. Surprised?

Well, here are the scientific facts, and this is the first surprise: Grass-fed meat is lower in total fats–but only bad fats. **Grass-fed meat has two to six times more omega-3 fatty acids than commercially fed meat.**[11-13]

Entire books have been written about EFAs, and the solid scientific studies are too numerous to mention. People who have ample amounts of omega-3s in their diet are less likely to have high blood pressure or an irregular heartbeat. Remarkably, they are also **50 percent less likely to suffer a heart attack.**[14]

I no longer know of many people who can afford to pass up a chance to improve brain function. Omega-3s are also essential for healthy brain cells. People who follow a diet rich in omega-3s are less likely to suffer from depression, schizophrenia, attention deficit disorder (hyperactivity) or Alzheimer's disease than those who are deficient in omega-3s.[14]

Extremely important to the readers of this book is that science shows that omega-3s may also reduce your risk of cancer. In animal studies, these essential fats have slowed the growth of a wide array of cancers and also kept them from spreading.[16,17] Since you need them anyway, even without a human study on cancer, I would recommend you take omega-3s.

Another benefit is that studies show recovery from surgery is more rapid when omega-3s are abundant in the diet.[17,18]

The higher the EFA content, the "fishier" the taste of the meat. In one study on range-fed (naturally fed) chicken, researchers found that adding a very small amount of natural vitamin E reduced the fishy flavor but maintained the EFAs.[13]

Escherichia coli (E. coli) is a real concern these days. One study found that cattle fed with commercial feeds passed on more *E. coli* that was resistant to stomach acid, while those fed hay for only five days had a dramatic reduction in the quantity and acid resistance of *E. coli.*[19]

Addressing the argument by commercial farmers that corn-fed cows produce more tender beef, it seems that may not be the case. Intramuscular fat (marbling fat) was studied, and researchers found "poor relationships between fat content and tenderness in commercially fed cows, which are high in saturated fat, and lean animals.[20] Tenderness can actually be manipulated via dietary supplements (EFAs and vitamin E) in feed. According to another study, flavor also improves in grass-fed lamb and beef as opposed to grain-fed animals.[21]

Omega-3s are most abundant in seafood and certain nuts and seeds such as flax seeds, walnuts and canola, but they are also found in animals and fish that feed as originally intended since omega-3s are formed in the chloroplasts of green leaves and algae.

(Remember Chapter 5 and what we learned about fish?)

When you buy an omega-3 supplement, be certain that you only buy one that can show third-party scientific validation that this oil is free of dioxin and PCBs but still active. While there is a patented distillation process that has been tested and can demonstrate these qualities, I cannot in this book make product recommendations by name, so I simply urge you to verify that data. Be wary, however, since every fish oil company claims theirs is clean, and that is not the case. If a company can demonstrate this third-party proof, they will be proud to show this proof to you. Otherwise, you should consider the oil toxic and stay away from it.

Now that we have discussed the nutritional value of food I would refer you to the three loss of nutrient charts on page (Plates 13 through 15).[7]

What You Need for Optimal Health
The list below shows what you need to achieve and maintain optimal health:
- Essential vitamins and minerals to create healthy cells
- Glyconutrients for cell-to-cell communication and immune support
- Phytonutrients to detoxify the system (plant nutrients)
- Phytohormones for glandular function (plant hormones)
- Essential fatty acids (EFAs) for cell regulation, hormonal function and metabolism
- Essential amino acids, which serve as the building blocks for all proteins
- Antioxidants to protect your cells from oxidative damage

Top-quality nutrients are no longer a luxury–they have become a necessity. As established in previous chapters, we cannot possibly eat enough food to get all the nutrients we need to fight the ravages of oxidative stress, the immune-lowering effects of psychological stress and the harm to our bodies caused by dietary stress.

There is excellent information already available on vitamins, minerals, essential fatty acids, amino acids and even phytonutrients, so I will not cover those to any great extent here. As for phytohormones, all your life you have unknowingly been consuming phytohormones periodically, if not daily, in the food you have eaten. But the subject of phytohormones is, in fact, so controversial that it requires a book in itself and will not be covered here.

Regarding antioxidants, the latest science shows that much of what we thought was true about them wasn't true at all. I will devote the following chapter to explaining their importance and not only what to do, but what to avoid. I will not merely repeat the outdated information you can see on any Web site or in a university textbook, nor will I be giving information based on gimmicks that have no scientific background but are designed to impress consumers. In addition, I will omit information based on superficial tests or the testing of only one antioxidant, or even multiple tests in Petri dishes. I will show you the latest third-party objective findings of how you can get the highest documented protection in your body, as tested in human blood.

But we do need to spend some time explaining the most promising new type of necessary nutrients yet identified–glyconutrients.

The Sugar Code of Life
The category of nutritional supplements called glyconutrients is so new that most of the experts in the use of dietary supplements still haven't heard of them or do not appreciate

their importance. Therefore, I will devote the remainder of this chapter to this subject.

As you will learn, glyconutrients occur naturally in many plants that have been used medicinally in various cultures for centuries. For example, aloe is recognized worldwide for its healing properties, but the functional component is actually a glyconutrient. The first glyconutrient complex made from many plants and sold as a dietary supplement that I am aware of became available to U.S. citizens back in 1996. Since then, several nutritional companies have jumped on the bandwagon.

You will soon learn that glyconutrients are not just one of the most recent discoveries, but without question, the most important for supporting human health. The word glyconutrient is derived from the Greek *"glyco"* meaning sweet. Some glyconutrients aren't very sweet, but they fall under the heading of a group of plant chemicals called saccharides. Saccharide is simply a chemical name for sugar. However, the word is important and will help you avoid confusing different sugars.

Generally speaking, when someone says the word "sugar," your first thought is something that tastes really good and is really bad for you. Sugar makes you fat or causes diabetes.[22,23] It is found in foods that you shouldn't eat because they contain table sugar. Table sugar is all too abundant. The average American adult consumes more than 75 lbs. (34.09kg) per year, and the average American child consumes 115 lbs. (52.27kg) per year. That's about 700 calories a day from sugar for each child. You will not do your child a favor by giving them anything with table sugar in it. According to the World Health Organization, diabetes is fast becoming the biggest single health issue in the world, and both you and your children should say no to foods that contain table sugar.

Table sugar is one of the principal causes of ill health, but there are necessary sugars without which you have virtually no hope for good health. The necessary glyconutrient sugars do not cause diabetes. They are essential nutrients and are very different from table sugar.

Let's cite another, more familiar analogy that might be helpful. Everyone knows that there are acids that are so caustic that if you put even one drop on steel, it could burn right through the metal. Now, that's obviously a bad acid. But there are also acids that are essential to your life. These are called amino acids. If you are deficient in certain essential amino acids, you will get sick and may die if they are not provided. Therefore, we can see that there are both good and bad acids.

Similarly, there are good sugars, and there are bad sugars. For those who prefer more specifics, let's address carbohydrates. Glyconutrients may be correctly referred to as carbohydrates, but once again, we must acknowledge that there are both good carbohydrates (glyconutrients) and bad carbohydrates, such as table sugar and foods that are high-glycolic. The bad carbohydrates make you fat, and, according to the U.S. National Institutes of Health (NIH), excess body fat is linked to at least 20 different diseases and illnesses.[23]

Good sugars (or good carbohydrates) are the same as glyconutritionals. They may be located in various science texts, articles and studies under any of the following names:
- **Biological sugars**
- **Monosaccharides (single sugars)**
- **Saccharides (sugars)**
- **Necessary sugars**
- **Necessary carbohydrates**

- Nutritional carbohydrates
- Glyconutrients (necessary sugars)

Let's get a few other definitions clear before we proceed to discuss the importance of glyconutrients:
- Glyconutrients–the eight known monosaccharides necessary for cell-to-cell communication
- Glyconutritional–a dietary supplement designed to provide glyconutrients
- Glycoproteins–glyconutrients bonded to proteins
- Glycoforms–any of several different glycosylated variants of a specified glycoprotein
- Glycosylated–the presence of one or more sugars added to a protein to form a glycoprotein
- Glycolipids–sugars joined to fats
- Glycoconjugates–broad term for all of the above

New Kid on the (Building) Blocks

Terms, like those above, under the heading of glyconutrients, may be something very new to you and your doctor. Glyconutrition is one of the newest areas of health science. Prior to 1965, there were no papers at all that discussed nutritional carbohydrates or glyconutrients. The only mention of sugars was either in the context of quick energy or about the negative effects of bad sugars (such as weight gain and diabetes). Since 1965, more than 20,000 papers have been written on glycoconjugates. Despite these documents, clinical trials and various individual studies, the majority of doctors have not yet heard the word "glyconutrients," nor do they understand why every human being needs them.

It's important to be realistic. The healthcare systems of all modern nations are driven by what is known as Western Biomedicine. Biomedicine may also be referred to as allopathic medicine. Allopaths are medical doctors–MDs. A medical doctor's training requires very high intelligence and a tremendous tenacity to survive the rigors of medical school, internship, etc. They are taught about drugs and surgery, but are not taught about dietary supplements to any great extent, if at all.

In fact, the vast majority of medical schools teach nothing or next to nothing on the therapeutic use of dietary supplements. Some doctors are taught that dietary supplements have no value, or perhaps are even dangerous.

You may wonder why this is the prevailing situation. The answer, I'm sad to say, comes down to money. Medical schools are sponsored in large part by pharmaceutical companies, and pharmaceutical companies have no interest in manufacturing and selling something that they cannot control financially. There is no profit motive for them to drive the knowledge of glyconutritionals or any other category of dietary supplements. Therefore, the vast majority of doctors are not aware of the information about glyconutritionals, and consequently the media also stays unaware since they get nearly all of their health-related information from medical doctors. This information gap leaves the general public in the dark about the most important nutritional breakthrough for their health yet (as of the time of this printing).

The discovery of the glyconutrient complex that I will discuss has now been patented in many countries around the world. Dozens more patents have been

filed in other countries and are currently pending. The pharmaceutical companies have spent countless millions researching individual <u>synthetic</u> saccharides, and in each case thus far they have failed. Although I have no psychic powers, I do not foresee a time when the pharmaceutical companies will create a synthetic saccharide that is better in all respects from safety to efficacy than what we find naturally occurring in plants. No pharmaceutical companies want to attempt to violate international patents on the glyconutritional complex. The fact that the big pharmaceutical companies are willing to spend millions in an attempt to create a synthesized version of even one glyconutrient speaks volumes about the general realization of their importance to human health in today's world.

Glycoconjugates have been discussed recently in a number of very important publications such as *Acta Anatomica,* an international peer review journal that devoted an entire issue to the glycosciences, or the study of glyconutrients. There is also a science journal called *Glycobiology,* devoted to this area. Studies have also been published in the well-known leading British medical journal, *The Lancet,* as well as many other scientific and lay publications.

In an issue of *Scientific American,* a magazine for both scientists and laymen, the cover story was "Sweet Medicine." One of the articles inside was titled "Saving Lives with Sugars."

From a scientific point of view, one of the most important documents to come out in the area of glyconutrients was the 1996 issue of *Harper's Biochemistry,* a medical biochemistry textbook.[24]

In this medical text, Robert Murray, MD, PhD, itemized the eight major monosaccharides known to be present in glycoproteins. He listed these saccharides as *glucose, galactose, mannose, fucose, xylose, N-acetyl-glucosamine, N-acetyl-galactosamine, and N-acetyl-neuraminic acid,* the latter also referred to frequently as either *NANA* or *sialic acid.*

Dr. Murray is eminently qualified to provide this information to medical students. He had a distinguished teaching and research career at the University of Toronto and has published over fifty scientific, peer-reviewed papers; authored multiple textbook articles; and been one of the authors of the last five editions of *Harper's Biochemistry.* He is working on the sixth as I am writing this second edition.

(A personal note: After meeting Dr. Murray in 1997, I have the honor to say we have become friends, and I have boundless personal respect for him as a scientist, teacher and man of high integrity).

How Much of a Very Good Thing?

How many glyconutrients do you need to eat in order to end up with the eight known necessary ones in your glycoproteins? Well, that is a question that hasn't been settled yet. Some experts believe that sugars behave differently than amino acids in many ways, not the least of which is in the digestive process. Until recently, the consensus among scientists in glycobiology was that since N-acetyl amino acids survive stomach acid, then N-acetyl saccharides would also do so.

However, other scientists believe that the N-acetyl saccharides often do not survive stomach acid well. Since there is too much at risk to take a chance, the most important thing to do would be to provide a complex of sugars that result in the N-acetyls being delivered to the cell surface receptors rather than just one that contains the N-acetyls and hope for the best.

If you get a product that has less than the full complex needed, you may not obtain complete function. However, to be fully objective, any product that offers even one of the above listed glyconutrients has value for your health and can make you feel better. The fact is if you have a health condition that requires only one additional saccharide, and you take a product with that one, your health will undoubtedly improve. The urgent question, however, is: Do you know if you need only one or two or five, or do you need the entire complex? You can't know at this point in time with the testing routinely available, and life is far too precious to take a chance on having less than you or your loved ones require for optimal health.

Ongoing research in glyconutrients is revealing more and more that herbals traditionally used to support immune function contain saccharides or glyconutrients that are also known to support immune function. Most of these plants have at least one glyconutrient, some have two or more, such as echinacea, various mushroom extracts and others. I cannot cover them all here, so I'll just offer a few examples.

Echinacea purpurea is a well-known herb traditionally used for symptoms related to the common cold. It is known to raise the count of white cells (immune cells) and has been found to contain a high amount of glyconutrients including galactose and arabinose, plus some uronic acids and the amino acids serine, alanine and *hydroxyproline* (if you are interested).[25]

One mushroom (*Pleurotus citrinopileatus*) being analyzed for anti-cancer properties in sarcoma 180 in mice was found to contain glucose, mannose, arabinose, galactose, xylose and fucose.[26] In one study on the hemagglutinating (blood clumping) activity of seven different mushrooms, numerous glyconutrients were isolated. Although more than one agglutinating factor was identified in the extracts, agglutination was partially inhibited nonspecifically by high concentrations of glucose, galactose, mannose, fucose and rhamnose.[27]

In other studies that were done to isolate and investigate the chemical structures of six different species of mushrooms (i.e. the *Basidiomycetes amanita virosa* {"death cup"}, *Calvatia exipuliformis* {"puffball"}, *Cantharellus cibarius* {"chanterelle"}, *Leccinum scabrum* {"red birch boletus"}, *Lentinus edodes* {Japanese shiitake}, and *Pleurotus ostreatus* {"oyster mushroom"}), the "glyco findings" (if you will) were mannose (attached to inositol) and fucose.[28,29]

In natural medicine mushrooms have been used for thousands of years for immune-related issues, but the users never knew they were using glyconutrients. The point is that plants that are known to have immune-supporting properties not coincidentally contain one or more glyconutrients.

One south sea island plant contains several glyconutrients and glycosides. Although this plant does not contain the entire complex I spoke of, it has one the highest number of glyconutrients I am aware of in a single plant. That plant is called *morinda citrifolia*, better known as "noni." It has some truly remarkable properties for the human immune system, including antitumor activity.[30,31] (A cautionary note here: The science of glycobiology doesn't get the attention or the research dollars it deserves, and there may be a plant as yet untested that has everything we need for health. I am simply relating what we know at the time of this printing.)

However, to have complete cell-to-cell communication and therefore complete cellular function, you still need to have all the glyconutrients required that result in the eight known essential saccharides for cell-to-cell communication. No single plant yet researched (at this time) contains all those glyconutrients. That is why a complete complex has been created from several different plant sources.

There are also many foods that contain one or more of these essential saccharides. Typically in the modern human diet we are getting two saccharides–glucose and galactose.[32,33] By the way, there is a popular myth that vegetarians are galactose-deficient since they don't eat dairy products. That's not correct. Even those people who avoid dairy still get galactose. While galactose is highest in dairy products, it's also found in various other foods, including some that are consumed by strict vegans. As for the other glyconutrient, glucose, an all-candy or all-bread diet would give you far too much of that glyconutrient.

As mentioned elsewhere in this book, it is a fact that our bodies were designed to live in a pristine world, free of synthetic toxins and other pollutants. It is also a fact that we were designed to eat raw, fresh, natural foods grown in soil with a high nutrient value. Thus it is entirely possible that our ancestors received the glyconutrients they needed from food each day–enough to cope with the conditions of their time. However, that world no longer exists, and the foods we eat provide much less nutrition (including glyconutrients) than most people (including many scientists) had supposed.[33]

The Glucose-only Theory–Fact or Fiction?

Recall the discussion earlier in this book about the recommendations by the National Academy of Sciences to double your daily intake of fresh fruits and vegetables, when almost no one is eating the earlier recommendation of 5-9 servings of fresh, raw fruits and vegetables to begin with. Also recall from earlier chapters that eating as many as ten servings of fresh raw fruits and vegetables would raise your protection against oxidative stress by a mere 13%.[34] How many servings are you willing to eat? How many can you afford to buy?

Scientists in the modern world have been hanging on to a very convenient theory. It's called the "glucose-only theory." This theory says that if you consume glucose, your body will go through an amazing and almost magical process of converting glucose via multiple enzymes into all of the necessary glyconutrients. If this theory were universally correct, it would be a great deal of fun. It means we could all eat candy and cupcakes and other forms of unhealthy foods, and by doing so improve our health. Most doctors in practice today were taught this glucose-only theory, and they don't know of the more recent research, which casts serious doubt on this concept.

In *The Journal of Pediatrics* (Nov. 1998), Dr. Hudson Freeze wrote that human ingestion studies show that mannose is readily absorbed and incorporated into glycoproteins via an active, independent pathway.[35] He too had been taught that if you consumed glucose, that glucose would turn into various other glyconutrients. But his observations showed that mannose (one of the most important glyconutrients for immune support) goes directly from your mouth into glycoproteins, exactly as your body was designed to have it done, through an independent pathway that never undergoes any conversion process. That information by itself, of course, is not sufficient to disprove the glucose-only theory. It only makes the theory seem somewhat suspicious.

Dr. Freeze further stated that, "Mannose for glycoprotein biosynthesis is assumed to come from glucose. Therefore, the finding that mannose–not glucose–corrects glycosylation defects was surprising." [35]

In December 1998, a radio-labeling study was done that added more strength to the argument that glucose-only always worked. In this study, radioactive isotopes were "tagged" to various substances so that they could be followed as they traveled through the bloodstream in order to see where they went and what they did. The scientists conducting this study tagged galactose, mannose and glucose. The study showed that galactose and mannose were directly incorporated into human glycoprotein without first being broken down into glucose. This result was a surprise. At least two of the eight known necessary sugars for cell-to-cell communication have their own pathways independent of glucose. The scientists concluded that glyconutrients could represent a new class of nutrients, just like vitamins, minerals, essential fatty acids and essential amino acids. [36]

In another study, published in March 1998 by Alton, et al., more data was compiled that began to disprove the glucose-only theory. This study showed that intact mannose molecules are rapidly absorbed from the intestines of rats into the blood, and mannose is cleared from the blood within hours. [37] The same study also showed that, contrary to prevailing wisdom, liver cells in tissue culture derive most of the mannose for glycoprotein synthesis directly from mannose, not from glucose. These experiments showed that mannose is absorbed, intact and unchanged, from the intestine into the blood, and then from the blood into the cells. These studies also indicated that dietary mannose may make a significant contribution to glycoprotein synthesis in mammals without glucose. The authors concluded, "This suggests that direct use of mannose is more important than conversion from glucose." So perhaps the all-cake-and-candy diet isn't all you need for health!

Let's look at just one more piece of evidence against the glucose-only theory. This theory assumes that all of us produce the enzymes we need every day in order to convert glucose into any of the known necessary saccharides. There are those doctors who believe that humans always produce sufficient enzymes either to fulfill the glucose-only theory or to simply transfer glyconutrients to their intended healthy destination.

Checking for Sugarprints

Whether the glucose-only theory really works or not, there is an unquestioned connection between disease processes in the diseases thus far tested and deficiencies of glyconutrients. In fact, one scientist has developed a method of testing for this connection that he calls "Sugar Printing."

This modern-day medical detective is one of the most respected researchers in the area of glycobiology. He is John S. Axford, BS, MD, FRCP (Fellow of the Royal College of Physicians). Dr. Axford serves on the editorial boards of three medical journals and on numerous medical and health-related committees. He is (at the time of printing) the immediate past-president of the Royal Society of Medicine, Section of Clinical Immunology and Allergy. Dr. Axford has authored, or co-authored, more than fifty published, peer-reviewed scientific papers, over one hundred published abstracts and letters, and two best-selling medical textbooks. He is actively involved with research in rheumatology and is especially interested in the glycobiology of arthritic diseases.

Dr. Axford studied the relationship of the enzyme that facilitates the transfer of the glyconutrient galactose to its intended destinations in rheumatoid disease, including rheumatoid arthritis (RA) and systemic lupus erythematosis (SLE). Dr. Axford observed that an enzyme called *galactosyltransferase* and the glyconutrient galactose were both lower in patients with RA and SLE than in the healthy people designated as "controls." He also noted that the severity of the disease was directly related to the degree of deficiency of galactose.[38,39]

Dr. Axford has been able to show that each rheumatic disease tested thus far with his sugar printing method has a unique "sugar print." Since 1965, a great deal has been studied regarding glyconutrients. However, at this point in time, very little is known about unlocking all of the secrets and codes. Dr. Axford's sugar printing isn't just interesting–it is extremely important and could someday lead to doctors being able to not only diagnose but also predict many diseases by the distinct print left by the presence or absence of the glyconutrients in the blood.

(Again on a personal note: I have been privileged to spend time with Dr. Axford, and my respect for him as a scientist is limitless. Dr. Axford is truly one of the current leaders in the world of scientific research.)

In the year 2000, scientists in London, England, presented facts about abnormal glycosylation and its relationship to disease at the Royal Society of Medicine Conference on Glycobiology and Medicine. It was, in my opinion, an appropriate way for progressive scientists to launch the new millennium.

At the time of this printing, ten rheumatic diseases have been studied, and in each case glyconutrients played a key role.

Abnormal Glycosylation
- Rheumatoid arthritis
- IgG abnormal, with reduced galactose levels
- Shape of molecule altered, inside exposed, altered immune recognition
- Severity of disease proportional to missing galactose
- Nine other rheumatic diseases associated with changes in sugar pattern
- Each disease tested had a unique sugar print

–RSM Conference, *Glycobiology and Medicine,* 2000[8]

As previously mentioned, Dr. Axford found that the severity of rheumatoid arthritis was directly proportional to the lack of galactose, one of the eight known necessary saccharides, and one of two saccharides that scientists tell us we get from our diet. These individuals clearly had too little of that glyconutrient, however. If unhealthy individuals can be documented to be deficient in one of the two glyconutrients we supposedly get in sufficient quantity from our diets, then what are the implications for those glyconutrients we get far too little of, and what of their enzyme connections?

Progress is definitely being made in the area of sugar printing, and most scientists who are aware of Dr. Axford's work eagerly anticipate the release of this technology for standard use in medical labs.

In *Journal of Pediatrics*, Dr. Freeze also tells us that there is very little information on the bioavailability of mannose in food, but he suspects that dietary mannose is probably insufficient to supply all glycosylation.[35] After an exhaustive review of the literature, Ramberg and McAnalley concluded that we are getting insufficient amounts of certain monosaccharides in our diets.[33]

Looking at the food chart (Plate 13),[33] we see the loss of saccharides following the processing of food. The blue bar represents the amount of saccharides of various types in a raw carrot. The yellow bar represents the amount of saccharides left in a cooked carrot. Some saccharides virtually disappear with cooking. What's very important to note is that the saccharides that make a carrot taste sweet are very high to begin with, and remain high even after cooking. Sucrose and glucose are not the healthiest sugars for you to eat in high quantities. Fructose, another sweet sugar, is healthful only at low levels. High levels of fructose do as much damage to health as high levels of sucrose.

The sugars that you need for cell-to-cell communication and immune modulation are predominantly *hexoses* (6c monosaccharides, meaning there are 6 carbon molecules) sugars along with the amino sugars *N-acetylglucosamine, N-acetylgalactosamine* and *N-acetylneuraminic acid,* which glycobiologists identify as a 9c sugar. If you are not a scientist, don't worry about it. I'm just endeavoring to be accurate. Although most human glycoprotein chains do not contain much *pentose* (xylose), xylose is still very important. As you see, on Plate 13 there are very small amounts of the hexose and pentose molecules present, compared to the sweet sugars like sucrose and glucose. Once the carrot has been cooked, there are virtually no hexose or pentose molecules left. That's because we are designed to eat raw carrots.

As I mentioned earlier, these saccharides are contained in many foods. However, there is no possibility of eating enough food daily to get the amounts of these saccharides needed to deal with the horrendous health threats, toxins and various other stresses discussed in this book. We have come to a time when, if you wish to maintain good health, and if you are to have any hope of fighting disease, you have to supplement various nutrients–vitamins, minerals, etc.–but you especially need to supplement glyconutrients.

How Cells Communicate

I've mentioned cell-to-cell communication several times. Let's discuss for a few moments why this is important. On the surface, the concept of cell-to-cell communication doesn't sound terribly interesting. However, let's construct a theoretical scenario in layman's terms to help demonstrate how important this process really is.

In your bloodstream you have an army that is ready to defend you, to protect you and to keep invaders from harming you. This army is made up of what are commonly called white blood cells. For our scenario we will use only the types of these cells that are known as lymphocytes–particularly T cells and B cells, both of which are critical to the action of the immune system. T cells directly attack disease-causing bacteria, viruses and toxins. They also regulate other parts of the immune system. B cells (the "scouts") produce antibodies that neutralize invaders or tag them for destruction by other agents of the immune system.

To keep this simple, let's continue our military example. The scout cell's job is to identify anything in your bloodstream that is not friendly and not healthful to you, such as an invading bacterium, virus or cancer cell. The scout cells can only do their job if they can communicate, and that requires sufficient glycosylation.

When these scout cells have been sufficiently glycosylated, they are able to recognize the enemy and tag it. Then they send a cell-to-cell communication (a signal) to T cell headquarters–the thymus gland, where T cells await their orders. If all of those cells are sufficiently glycosylated, immune system headquarters will then send a communication to the soldier cells of the body. The soldiers leave immune system headquarters to search out and destroy any cell that has been tagged by the scout cells.

If these scout cells do NOT have complete glycoproteins, they will be unable to differentiate a friendly cell from an unhealthy and unfriendly one. These scout cells might tag or stamp healthy cells. The soldier cells of the body, which simply follow orders, locate any tagged cell, then attack and destroy it. This happens in autoimmune diseases in humans when one's own immune system is attacking itself. It starts with a miscommunication.

This is an oversimplification of the process. But there are, as I have mentioned, other agents of the immune system. Of course, this book is not an immunology text. Besides the autoimmune scenario I just mentioned, scout cells that do not have complete glycoproteins might also fail to recognize dangerous cells and therefore not tag them. In this case, the soldier cells would do nothing, and allow enemy cells to cause infection or disease. This is the first part of what happens when an immune system fails to respond to a challenge. The affected individual would continue to get more and more ill, and perhaps in some cases, even die.

There are myriad factors to ensure good health, and no nutrient stands alone. But clearly without cell-to-cell communication, you have no hope for good health because without communication (or signaling), there can be no function.

Every Day Should be a "Glyco-Day"

Everything you've learned thus far about so-called alternative medicine (or what I prefer to call complementary medicine) you've learned with a Western biomedicine thought process. For instance, take the use of herbal medicine. As the name implies, this is when an herbal substance is used as a medicine. You have a symptom. You take the herbal for relief of the symptom. When you help support your body with that herbal (which is far less toxic than pharmaceutical drugs), your body–as long as it receives everything else it needs–can respond to the challenge and defend, heal and restore you.

Vitamins and minerals are essential for the process of assembling healthy cells as well as many other functions of the body, but glyconutrients and their corresponding proteins are essential for cell-to-cell communication. If your cells cannot communicate, you have no function and, therefore, no hope. It's that simple and explains why glyconutri-

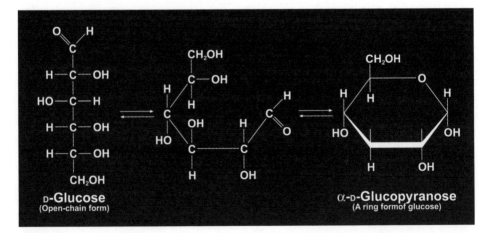

D-Glucose
(Open-chain form)

α-D-Glucopyranose
(A ring form of glucose)

Plate 1

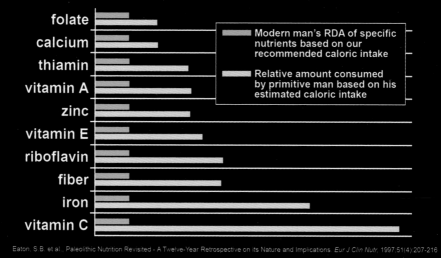

Comparison Between Primitive and Modern Man's Intake of Some Vitamins, Minerals and Fiber*

folate
calcium
thiamin
vitamin A
zinc
vitamin E
riboflavin
fiber
iron
vitamin C

■ Modern man's RDA of specific nutrients based on our recommended caloric intake

■ Relative amount consumed by primitive man based on his estimated caloric intake

Eaton. S.B. et al., Paleolithic Nutrition Revisited - A Twelve-Year Retrospective on its Nature and Implications. *Eur J Clin Nutr*, 1997;51(4):207-216

Plate 2

Loss of Antioxidant Nutrients When a Carrot is Cooked

mg nutrient per 100g carrot

vitamin C
vitamin A
tocopherols
vitamin E activity
manganese
zinc

0   1   2   3   4   5   6   7

■ raw carrot
■ cooked carrot

Souci. S.W., et al., *Food Composition and Nutrition Tables*. Boca Raton, FL: CRC Press, 2000.

Plate 3

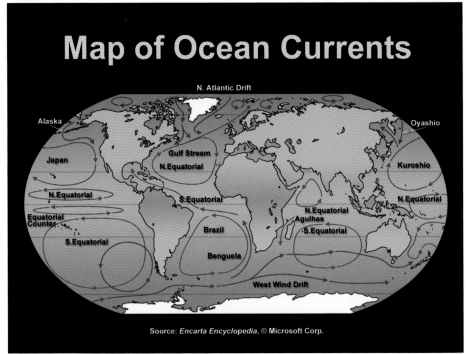

Map of Ocean Currents

Source: *Encarta Encyclopedia*, © Microsoft Corp.

Plate 4

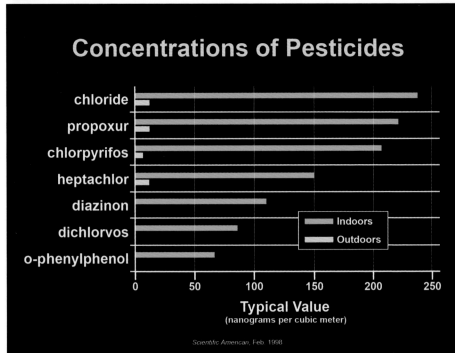

Concentrations of Pesticides

Scientific American, Feb. 1998

Plate 5

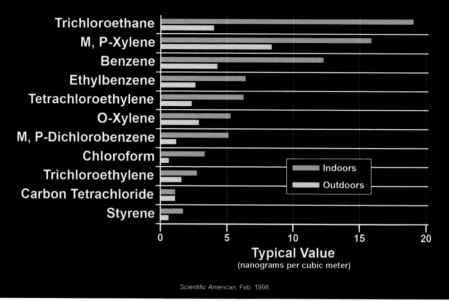

Volatile Organic Compounds

Trichloroethane	
M, P-Xylene	
Benzene	
Ethylbenzene	
Tetrachloroethylene	
O-Xylene	
M, P-Dichlorobenzene	
Chloroform	
Trichloroethylene	
Carbon Tetrachloride	
Styrene	

Indoors
Outdoors

0   5   10   15   20

Typical Value
(nanograms per cubic meter)

Scientific American, Feb. 1998

Plate 6

Toxins in Your Home

Everyday toxins: You're better off outdoors	Respirable Particles (µg/cubic meter)	Toxic, Volatile, Organic Compounds (µg/cubic meter)
Exposure	0 100 200 300	1 10 10^2 10^3 10^4
Photocopier with dry toner *(formaldehyde, styrene, etc.)*		
Room with smokers *(benzene, many others)*		
Carpeted home *(pesticides, many others)*		
Steamy bathroom *(chloroform)*		
Drycleaning in closet *(perchloro-, trichloro-ethane)*		
Enclosed parking garage *(benzene, many others)*		
Fireplace *(benzene, many others)*		
Kitchen fumes *(many different components)*		
Household cleaners *(paradichlorobenzene, many others)*		
Outdoors in the city *(many different components)*		
Outdoors in the suburbs *(many different components)*		

Ott and Roberts. Everyday Exposure to Toxic Pollutants, *Scientific American*, 278(2):86-91. 1998

Plate 7

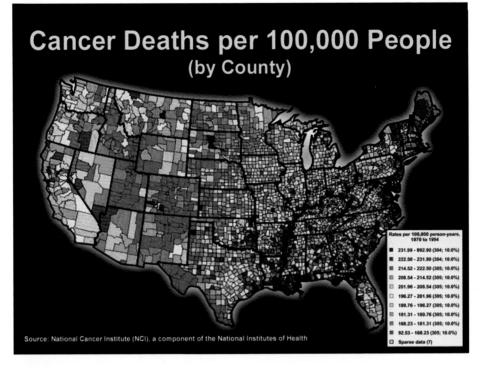

Plate 8

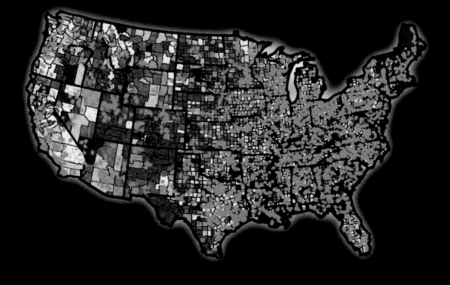

Plate 9

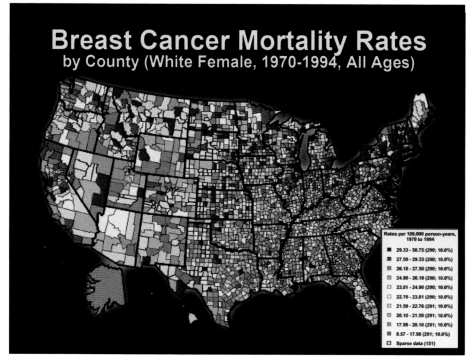

Breast Cancer Mortality Rates
by County (White Female, 1970-1994, All Ages)

Rates per 100,000 person-years, 1970 to 1994

- 29.33 - 50.75 (290; 10.0%)
- 27.50 - 29.33 (290; 10.0%)
- 26.18 - 27.50 (290; 10.0%)
- 24.90 - 26.18 (290; 10.0%)
- 23.81 - 24.90 (290; 10.0%)
- 22.76 - 23.81 (290; 10.0%)
- 21.59 - 22.76 (291; 10.0%)
- 20.10 - 21.59 (291; 10.0%)
- 17.98 - 20.10 (291; 10.0%)
- 8.57 - 17.98 (291; 10.0%)
- Sparse data (151)

Plate 10

Emissions Distribution Map
Air Pollutants

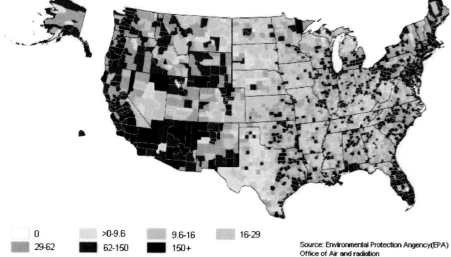

- 0
- 29-62
- >0-9.6
- 62-150
- 9.6-16
- 150+
- 16-29

Source: Environmental Protection Angency(EPA)
Office of Air and radiation

Plate 11

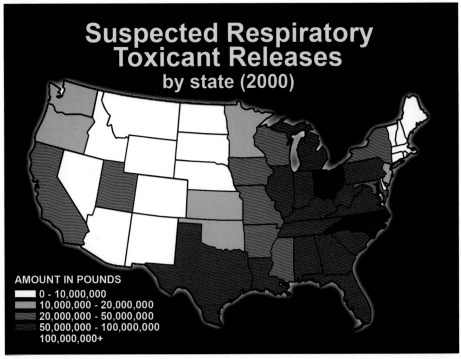

Plate 12

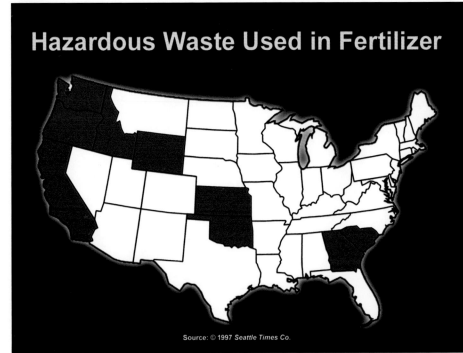

Plate 13

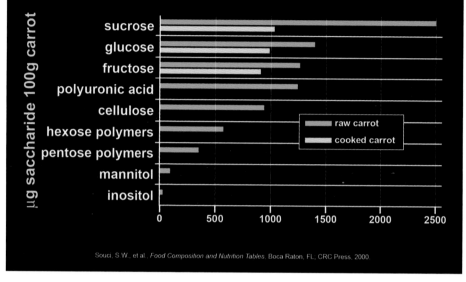

Loss of Saccharides Following Food Processing

μg saccharide 100g carrot

- sucrose
- glucose
- fructose
- polyuronic acid
- cellulose
- hexose polymers
- pentose polymers
- mannitol
- inositol

Legend: raw carrot, cooked carrot

X-axis: 0, 500, 1000, 1500, 2000, 2500

Souci, S.W., et al., *Food Composition and Nutrition Tables*, Boca Raton, FL; CRC Press, 2000.

Plate 14

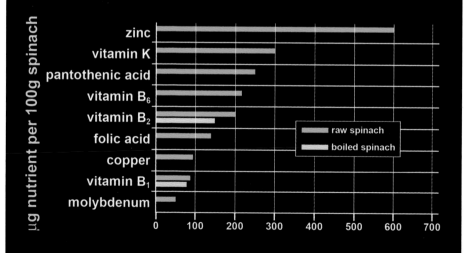

Loss of Vitamins and Minerals Following Cooking of Spinach

μg nutrient per 100g spinach

- zinc
- vitamin K
- pantothenic acid
- vitamin B$_6$
- vitamin B$_2$
- folic acid
- copper
- vitamin B$_1$
- molybdenum

Legend: raw spinach, boiled spinach

X-axis: 0, 100, 200, 300, 400, 500, 600, 700

Plate 15

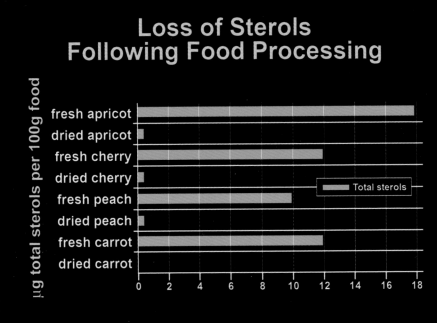

ents were the most important health discovery of the 20th century, and remains the most important nutritional foundation for human health in the 21st century.

Your doctor was probably taught that cell-to-cell communication was facilitated through amino acids. Since leaving medical school, most doctors haven't learned otherwise.

The problem is that amino acids can link in only two ways. A and B can link as AB or BA. But glyconutrients are what biologists call ring structures. They have a carbon backbone with O (oxygen) and H (hydrogen) molecules attached. This allows sugars to link with a virtually infinite variety of combinations. This process is also the only thing that can facilitate cell-to-cell communication since it's the only way you can spell virtually every "word" necessary to communicate from one cell to another.

Glyconutrients have (refer to chart on preceding page):
• Ring structures
• Carbon backbone with O and H attached
• An infinite variety of combinations

Once again, something taught in medical school until very recently has now been shown to be incorrect. This is not your doctor's fault. Don't expect your doctor to keep up with every change that occurs. Your doctor is extremely busy. He or she is inundated with publications and journals. Each year more than a quarter of a million pages of information on dietary supplements alone are published in scientific articles. No human being can possibly keep up with that. It is not your doctor's fault that he or she doesn't know this information yet. Showing them this book can help them get current in the 21st century for their patients.

Let me emphasize this in a different way. It doesn't matter what kind of cell you are talking about–brain cell, liver cell, kidney cell, immune cell, reproductive cell, a cell in your eye, a cell in your skin–all cells in your body require the same eight known necessary saccharides or glyconutrients and for the same reason–cell-cell communication, as well as many other important functions.

You cannot be sure if you have all eight glyconutrients where you need them at all times. No matter who you are, where you live, your age, your sex or state of health, glyconutrients in my opinion must be part of your daily health plan if you wish to achieve and maintain optimal health.

Glyconutrients are absolutely essential for:
• Normal cellular processes
• Cellular immunity
• Recognition and response
• Antibody function
• Signaling and recruitment

Ongoing research continues to support the concept that glyconutrients are vital in all functions. At the time of this printing, scientists had confirmed at least twelve congenital defects of glycosylation (CDG).[35] **A very wide range of effects (including death) have been seen where glycosylation is not complete. The heart-rending and mysterious disorder called sudden infant death syndrome or SIDS, also known as crib death, is now known to be one of these defects. They go undiagnosed most of the time since doctors are not trained in glyconutrients and would never think to**

look in this direction for an answer. Something as simple as a missing glyconutrient can trigger tragic miscommunication of cells.

Congenital Defects of Glycosylation
- First reported in 1980
- At least twelve now recognized (at the time of this printing)
- Range of clinical outcomes include death
- Vast majority go undiagnosed
- Contribute to many unexplained illnesses, including SIDS (crib death)
  –RSM Conference, Glycobiology & Medicine, 2000[38]

> **"Glyconutritionals–including mannose, fucose and glucose–have been documented to be therapeutic and even life-saving."**
> –RSM Conference, *Glycobiology & Medicine*, 2000[38]

In certain cases, glyconutritionals have been confirmed to correct the abnormal glycoproteins in congenital defects of glycosylation. That is extremely good news. There are cases that go undiagnosed and problems, which have been diagnosed as genetic, that doctors typically consider beyond help. **Here we have science to show that adding glyconutritionals can correct a number of these congenital defects. There is more hope now than anyone had ever before dreamed of.**

The twelve defects so far discovered (there will certainly be more) are only the beginning, the tip of the iceberg. Congenital defects of glycosylation should be considered in every patient, including children, who have unexplained clinical conditions. Besides the sites I have listed below, using keywords on an Internet search such as cross-referencing glyconutrients and CDGs will give you some valuable hits.

Other excellent sources for information about CDGs are *cdgs.com* and Online Mendelian Inheritance in Man, OMIMTM.40 Also highly recommended are McKusick-Nathans Institute for Genetic Medicine, Johns Hopkins University (Baltimore, MD) and the National Center for Biotechnology Information, National Library of Medicine (Bethesda, MD), 2000, *http://www.ncbi.nlm.nih.gov/omim/*

Glyconutrients and Major Health Issues
From scientific data thus far, we know that glyconutrients are important in the following:
- Asthma–mannose and N-acetyl galactosamine[41]
- Allergies such as contact dermatitis–fucose[42]
- Bronchial anaphylaxis–NANA[43]
- Cases of cancer–mannose, fucose, glucosamine and galactose[44]
- Various inflammations–N-acetyl galactosamine and N-acetyl glucosamine[45]
- Infections–mannose and NANA[46]
- Malaria–NANA[47,48]

Doctors, understandably, are cautious when looking at any kind of a nutritional substance that they do not understand. This is why progressively more educational materials are being made available. However, as the old saying goes, "You can lead a horse to water, but you can't make him drink."

Doctors are accustomed to seeing things that affect the immune system in ways that either stimulate or suppress. What they are not used to seeing in the pharmaceutical world are natural chemicals designed to help the body achieve its own balance, or homeostasis.

For example, glycoproteins on cell surface proteins of endothelial cells are involved in the control of transplant rejection. This is a very controversial area. Most doctors know that there is reliable information available showing that glyconutrients improve immune function. But physicians remain very cautious, when transplant patients come to them with the concept of taking glyconutrients, doctors typically respond, "Don't take them. They are immune stimulants."

However, glyconutrients have been shown to be immune modulators, not immune stimulants. An immune modulator is something that causes the immune system to achieve balance, not to always be stimulated or suppressed.

Let's look at two examples:

Lupus erythematosus is an autoimmune disorder where the immune system is working too high and against itself. Chronic fatigue and fibromyalgia are conditions in which the immune system is low and needs a boost. In both cases, individuals taking glyconutrients have had their health improve in virtually all of the markers.[49-51] This indicates that for autoimmune problems, the immune system must be modulated downward. And with immune problems, the immune system must be modulated upward to achieve balance. Balance is the only true state of wellness.

Help Educate Your Doctor

Having said that, I urge you not to self-diagnose or self-prescribe. Get your doctor involved with this process. Remember: Serious and even fatal disorders sometimes go undiagnosed because the vast majority of doctors have not been educated in this area. You can be the first to bring glyconutrients to your doctor's attention.

Oh, I know you're going to say, "Well, my doctor won't listen," or, "My doctor said no." Well, I would remind you of two things: One–if you're not an expert on something, you have no business giving advice. So is that doctor who said no trained in glyconutrient therapies? Two–if your doctor won't listen, find a new doctor who will. If your doctor's ego is more important to him or her than finding answers for your health, then you don't want to waste any more time with that doctor.

As far as I am concerned, there are at the time of this printing 6.5 billion human beings who need glyconutrients. I feel they should be a part of everyone's daily health support. In conditions where individuals are in very serious health situations, you may want to talk with a doctor specifically trained in glyconutrients. Transplant patients would be one example. They are obviously very compromised, or they wouldn't have needed the transplant to begin with. These individuals may die from any number of complications involved in transplants. Your doctor cannot make an informed decision unless he or she has been informed. If the doctor handling your transplant has not been educated in that area, he or she can go to *GlycoScience.org*, learn about immune modulation and safety with glyconutrients, and then link to other areas if he or she is open to learning more about it. Decisions of this type should involve a doctor trained in glyconutrients.

Leukocytes, endothelial cells, fibroblasts and other cells that contribute to the innate immune system via phagocytosis are regulated by glycoproteins. Adaptive immune effectors are also glycosylated.[96] And we know that complete glycoproteins are essential for wound healing and in cancer, inflammation and other clinical conditions involving cell growth and cell death.[39]

Doctors must necessarily be cautious with their patients, especially where there is a life-threatening disease. Doctors typically say to their patients who ask about glyconutri-ents, "Don't take them." They rarely give an explanation because they do not understand them, but they don't want their patients to know they don't understand glyconutrients. Again, your doctor cannot make an educated decision unless he or she has been informed.

Some doctors have already taken that bold step into what is for them unknown terri-tory. They have found that glyconutrients are essential in all matters of cellular function, including cancer. Dr. Glen Hyland (an oncologist) did a pilot survey of 127 patients. One hundred completed the survey, and he found that not only were glyconutrients not harmful, but also in cases that would not have otherwise responded to chemotherapy or radiation, these patients did recover.[52] That means the glyconutrients were vital! What follows is a portion of Dr. Hyland's pilot survey.

Responses to Dietary Supplementation While Undergoing Cancer Treatment
One hundred cancer patients gathered from a three-state area had modern dietary supplements added to their diets while undergoing standard radiation or chemotherapy. The results were reported by Dr. Hyland as listed below:

1. Standard treatment was not neutralized by dietary supplements containing antioxidants and micronutrients.
2. Radiation and chemotherapy effects against tumor cells were more effective.
3. Normal cells (bone marrow, liver, kidney and mucosal basal cells) were protected from treatment damage.
4. Malignancies not responsive to therapy, i.e. sarcomas, responded to the combina-tion.
5. Quality of life while having treatment was improved significantly.

–G. Hyland, 1999[52]

Can you see the wonderful health implications of this study? Dr. Hyland found that the quality of life of those patients was dramatically improved with no cell damage to healthy cells and greatly reduced negative effects of the chemotherapy and radiation.

Another paper is so noteworthy regarding cancer that I am compelled to quote the entire abstract.

"An elderly woman with adenocarcinoma of the colon was treated with standard thera-pies (surgery, radiation and chemotherapy). She demonstrated exceptional tolerance to treat-ments. This individual took 2-4g of glyconutritional supplements once or twice daily since her diagnosis. This report covered two years, during which she was treated with IV 5-FU twice, and oral and topical 5-FU once each. She experienced only mild diarrhea and fatigue follow-ing the final two rounds of 5-FU therapy, and no other expected adverse effects, such as hair loss, mouth ulcerations or nausea and vomiting. This lady also recovered quickly from colon surgery and tolerated radiotherapy with no adverse effects. The remarkable tolerance to can-cer therapy seen in this patient serves to demonstrate the role nutrition may play in enhanc-ing the quality of life of cancer patients." [53]

Can you imagine cancer therapy with fewer adverse effects, including hair loss, mouth ulcerations and nausea and or vomiting? If you have cancer, what could be better than tolerating the treatments with reduced adverse effects? Glyconutrients

may provide the most complementary strategy for supporting modern medicine!

According to Dr. John Axford and other scientists attending the Royal Society of Medicine Symposium, many proteins are glycosylated. There is, however, far too little information on glycobiology available in medical textbooks, and many major diseases involve glycoconjugates.

Now that you've learned what glyconutrients are and their importance to your health, the question remains: How much do you take? That's not as simple as you might think. Most people have been conditioned in the modern world with a drug mentality. As an example, if you have a bacterial infection, you might be prescribed to take an antibiotic, let's say at 500mg three times a day for 10 days. That is an average based on scientific study. The pharmaceutical will work on a biochemical reaction or system and be far more predictable than a natural substance. However, unexpected reactions to properly prescribed pharmaceutical drugs, not doctor error, are the fourth- leading cause of death in North America. Even pharmaceutical drugs—synthetic and highly predictable—are not fully predictable in terms of dose and time.

Therefore, how can we expect a food to be dosed precisely?

Glyconutrients are necessary for every cell of your body. It would be nice if all of your cells were born at the same moment and died on a given predictable moment. But that's not the way it works. When you take glyconutrients orally, you are attempting to maintain the glycosylation of all of the cells of your body.

Cells are constantly being born and dying. Your trillions of cells have different life spans. Some of them, as you can see on the cell chart, live for hours and some live for years, and virtually every time period in-between.[54]

Life Spans of Some Cells of the Human Body

Cell Type	Life Span
Granulocytes: eosinophils basophils, neutrophils	10 hours-3 days
Stomach lining cells	2 days
Sperm cells	2-3 days
Colon cells	3-4 days
Epithelia of small intestine	1 week or less
Platelets	10 days
Skin epidermal cells	2-4 weeks
Lymphocytes	2 months to more than a year (highly variable)
Red blood cells	4 months
Macrophages	months-years
Endothelial cells	months-years
Pancreas cells	1 year or more
Bone cells	25-30 years

We cannot predict which cells will receive their full, necessary complement of glyconutrients, nor can we predict how many will get the glyconutrients they need with each dose taken. It is theoretically possible to take an oral dose of glyconutrients, supply 500,000 cells with the glyconutrients they need, and have 100,000 of those cells continue to live on while 400,000 of them have expired. The expired cells are being replaced by cells that also need the necessary glyconutrients, and you may or may not have sufficient glyconutrients available at that moment to get the job done.

Many glycoproteins have a half-life of 10 days or fewer, so they are built up and degraded in quite a short time. However, a continual, ongoing supply of glyconutrients may be essential to be used for new glycoprotein synthesis. With this fact in mind, in at least some cases it will take months of having a sufficient and steady supply of completely glycosylated glycoproteins to resolve, or begin to resolve, your particular health issue. With this same idea in mind, it is important to take glyconutrients—not just like you would take a drug for a certain number of days or until you feel well, but every day for the rest of your life.

In my experience the other key issue is what I call your body's "threat priority list." This is a theory of mine, not a rigorously tested scientific fact. However, I believe it is true due to many years of clinical observation. But without the funding for proper research, it remains just a theory.

Okay, so what is the body's "threat priority list?" I have observed that the body will, if it is functioning correctly (and that is key), work on whatever it thinks is most important to your health. You may recall that various diseases can progress simultaneously in the human body, and the individual with them may be totally unaware. Breast cancer was the example I used earlier. I chose that example because most people know someone, knew someone, or will know someone with breast cancer.

After their breast cancer has been diagnosed, those individuals will tell you that they had felt fine. They were symptom-free of the breast cancer for the 5 to 30 years it took for the breast cancer to form in their body. It is possible, for example, that someone might have fibromyalgia, which they are painfully aware of. They also may have breast cancer brewing in their body. Of course, they will be unaware of the breast cancer, and until it reaches a certain point, it cannot be diagnosed.

With this in mind, they may take glyconutrients daily, and their fibromyalgia will not seem to improve. What may be happening in this case is a shifting of glyconutrients by the body to the fight against a more serious foe, and little or none is helping the condition of fibromyalgia, which is an agonizing—but not life-threatening—condition.

Your body's first priority is keeping you alive, not keeping you comfortable.

For more than eight years, I've seen individuals with fibromyalgia who experienced a quality of life enhancement in a matter of days. I've also seen some cases where it took months before they experienced the same level of enhancements. I strongly suspect in those cases that something more serious was going on in their bodies than they were aware of or could be diagnosed. You could create that same theoretical scenario with virtually any type of illness.

So, how long should it take to see results? Many people will take glyconutrients for the first few days and have tremendous and seemingly miraculous results. Many will not. This is because we are each biochemically and genetically unique. Glyconutrients are food—not—drugs and we cannot therefore predict the time as you would have with drugs. We are used to a doctor diagnosing a problem prescribing a synthetic drug and saying, "Well for this situation 1 pill three times a day for ten days" as an example.

In order for your body to do what is what designed to do for your health, it must have the tools it was designed to have. All cells have different lifespans and there

is no way to predict which cells will be glycosylated with any given serving of glyconutrients.[54] To complicate matters some cells have a glycosylation have life of as little as ten days. For this reason I recommend everyone use glyconutrients as part of their daily health plan for their entire life's. Don't think of them as a drug to get rid of symptoms but rather as part of a new lifestyle plan to support optimal wellness the rest of your life. With this in mind I have some recommendations below in terms of amounts and time but keep in mind they are general.

My Recommendations

It is optimal for you to cleanse your body before you start taking glyconutrients. I say optimal, but this doesn't mean that you can't receive nutritional benefits from taking glyconutrients before you've done a system cleanse. My system cleansing recommendations are as follows:

Mild general system cleanse

1. Eat very light or fast. Heavy meals–especially if they are heavy in protein–inhibit system detoxification.
2. Your diet should consist of only fresh, raw fruits and vegetables during the cleansing. No cooked foods.
3. If you choose to "juice fast," do so only under a doctor's supervision.
4. Fast only under supervision of a doctor experienced in this area.
5. Drink a minimum of 8 eight-ounce glasses of water daily. Preferably, sip water all day.
6. Use distilled water while detoxifying, but never for more than for two weeks consecutively.
7. A system cleanse should take between 2 and 14 days, depending how toxic your body has become.
8. Use filtered or reverse osmosis water the rest of the year.
9. At least one of those glasses needs to have the juice of 1/4 fresh lemon squeezed into it. Preferably up to four glasses.
10. Add 10 grams of soluble fiber once daily before bed. The fiber can be oat or psyllium.
11. A doctor knowledgeable in this area will often recommend nutrients to supplement the cleansing process. These may include:
    - A daily multiple vitamin/mineral supplement
    - Milk thistle
    - Beetroot powder
    - Dandelion root powder
    - A phytonutrient supplement
    - SAM-e (s-adenosylmethionine)

The above recommendations are for a general mild system cleanse. Liver, gallbladder and parasite cleanses are more severe and not pertinent to this book.

Maximum benefits will occur if you do a system cleanse first. Otherwise, you should expect to have some detoxification reactions. Those toxins that I spoke of are accumulating in your body in very tiny amounts each hour of every day, no matter where you live. These are going into your body in such tiny amounts that unless your system is extremely compromised, you will be unlikely to notice any symptoms associated with those toxins. However, remember that besides the benefits of cell-to-cell communication and immune modulation, glyconutrients have been shown in *in vitro* studies to raise glutathione levels.[55,56] Glutathione not only acts as an antioxidant in your blood but will cause your body to increase its detoxification reactions.

As your body begins to rid itself of chemical toxins, you may experience symptoms associated with those toxins. You might have skin rashes, headaches, nausea, malaise, depression, fatigue and gastrointestinal distress–any of those symptoms known to be associated with the more than 75,000 synthetic chemicals in our environment today. If you do a system cleanse before you begin taking glyconutrients, you are less likely to have any detoxification experiences or symptoms at all. I strongly recommend that you consult with a doctor who has training and experience in glyconutrients to help you understand how best to use glyconutrients considering your personal condition and overall health.

There is a paper on glyconutritional safety that just might be useful to share with your physician. This paper has a table with safety information for each individual sugar.[57] That's pretty handy when you want to convince your doctor that glyconutrients are safe.

In general, a healthy individual who is not using additional antioxidant support but is otherwise apparently healthy and symptom-free may begin with as little as 0.44 grams taken twice daily. It is extremely important to take glyconutrients at least twice daily: 0.44 grams translates to approximately a quarter of a teaspoon. For most people, this will not be enough in my opinion and, as the threats to our health from myriad sources discussed in this book increase, health support of all types (not just glyconutrients) may have to be increased daily.

Healthy people need minimal supplemental support, but the greater the health challenges, the more support you may need. For those with minor health issues, I recommend slightly more nutritional support. Take a minimum of 0.88 grams twice daily; 0.88 grams translates to approximately half of a teaspoon.

I recommend even more nutritional support for those with significant health issues or who have been chronically ill. They should start with 1.76 grams (a full teaspoon) twice daily for at least 90 days, but preferably for 180 days. Keep cellular turnover in mind. You need to give your body the time to get your cells sufficiently glycosylated. Don't start on glyconutrients, take them for only a few days and then quit because you haven't gotten the results that you expected.

If I were still in practice, I would probably recommend 1.76 grams or one full teaspoon twice daily for every new patient for at least 120 days since there may be things going on in them that we cannot yet diagnose. As Ben Franklin said, "An ounce of prevention is worth a pound of cure." In the 21st century, I think an ounce of prevention is worth a metric ton of cure!

If you suffer from a degenerative free radical disease, you should consider at least 10.56 grams to 15.84 grams twice daily, which translates to approximately 2 to 3 tablespoons twice daily for at least 90 but preferably 180 days.

While I was in practice, I learned many things about the use of glyconutrients besides their benefits. There was never a shortage of patients coming to see me with serious health challenges. Often, where time was of the essence, I needed to find out if there were any patterns in changing the recommended amounts in terms of time. Two things I always want to avoid are failure when a patient needs help and costing them more money than necessary.

I found over many months of trial and error using traditional allopathic methods for documentation–such as serum (blood) analysis and urinalysis–that there was a discernible pattern in most cases. When people are desperate and time really counts, they want to know how much, how long, and what is the maximum they can consume to get the quickest results. Well, I have already discussed amounts. (Please remember that those are only general guidelines, not specific individual prescriptions.)

As for time, these were my general findings: It was very rare to be able to document any beneficial changes in fewer than 72 hours at any levels I tried. The average time required for changes, which I could document, was typically around seven days for matters related to the body. So, if you follow the general amounts as recommended above, then seeing specific changes in fewer than 72 hours wouldn't make sense in most cases.

For severe problems, such as those listed above, you should increase by 1.76 grams every seven days. For problems related to brain chemistry, no fewer than 10 days, but more on the average of 14 days. For example, you would add an additional 1.76 grams every fourteen days until the benefits you seek could be documented. Glyconutrients are not toxic, and experiments have been done with as much as 100 grams daily, although I am not advocating those levels. I am simply stating that the minimum of 0.44 grams twice daily is just that–a minimum, not a maximum.

I want to reinforce strongly, as I have already mentioned, that you should not self-diagnose or self-prescribe. A patient needs a thorough examination to arrive at a diagnosis and to develop a therapeutic program using any type of substances. Guesswork is not acceptable as far as I am concerned. I strongly recommend you find a health professional who is trained in the use of glyconutrients or who is willing to learn about them. The information above is general and not meant to replace the care or advice of a doctor who is trained in the use of glyconutrients. If your doctor isn't trained in the science and use of glyconutrients, he or she has no factual basis for giving you advice on their use.

Glyconutrients are unique because they are needed for virtually every cell of the body and although they are not medicines, without them the body cannot perform the functions it was designed to perform. Hundreds of benefits have already been documented, from addressing everything from stress to cancer.[58]

The human body will correct itself, but only if it has the tools to do the job it was designed to do.

Some Final Thoughts on Glyconutrients
- During the early 20th century, carbohydrates were thought to be compounds used to provide energy without any other functions.
- In the first years of the 21st century, we have learned that necessary carbohydrates in the form of glyconutrients are vital for correct structure, function, relationships of cells, membranes, messenger molecules, enzymes, antibodies, hormones, binding, signaling, tumor spread and all other biological systems.
- Modern diets are deficient in glyconutrients, as well as other nutrients.
- Growing evidence of the value of glyconutrients has been documented in human, animal and cell biology studies.
- Even congenital defects of glycosylation have shown improvement with glyconutrients.
- Glyconutrients are modulators, not stimulators.
- Many diseases relate to abnormal glycobiology.
- Many diseases related to abnormal glycobiology go unrecognized.
- Research shows some diseases can be sugar-printed.
- What we have learned thus far is only the tip of the iceberg.

References

1. Rayman MP, Rayman MP. The argument for increasing selenium intake. *Proc Nutr Soc.* 2002;61(2):203-215.
2. UNICEF and the Micronutrient Initiative. *Vitamin and Mineral Deficiency: A Global Progress Report.* March 24, 2004: www.unicef.org/media/files/vmd.pdf
3. Arthur JR, Nicol F, Beckett GJ. Selenium deficiency, thyroid hormone metabolism, and thyroid hormone deiodinases. *Am J Clin Nutr.* 1993;57(2 Suppl):236S-239S.
4. Arthur JR. The role of selenium in thyroid hormone metabolism. *Can J Physiol Pharmacol.* 1991;69(11):1648-1652.
5. Fletcher. *Modern Miracle Men.* Paper presented to the 74th Session of U.S. Senate, June 5, 1936.
6. Bergner, Paul. *The Healing Power of Minerals, Special Nutrients and Trace Elements.* Prima Publishing, Rocklin, CA 1997
7. Ramberg J, McAnalley B. From the farm to the kitchen table: A review of the nutrient losses in foods. *GlycoScience & Nutrition* 2002;5(3):1-12.
8. NUTRACON: The Event for Nutraceuticals, Natural Products, Services & Sources. July 9-11, 2001, San Diego, California
9. Mayer A-M. Historical changes in the mineral content of fruits and vegetables. *Brit Food J.* 1997; 96: 207-211.
10. Guynup S. Arctic life threatened by toxic chemicals, groups say. *National Geographic Today.* October 8, 2002.
11. Fukumoto GK, Kim YS, Oduda D, Ako H. Chemical composition and shear force requirement of loin eye muscle of young, forage-fed steers. *Research Extension Series.* 1995;161:1-5.
12. Koizumi I, Suzuki Y, et al. Studies on the fatty acid composition of intramuscular lipids of cattle, pigs and birds. *J Nutr Sci Vitaminol* (Tokyo). 1991; 37(6):545-554.
13. Wood JD, Enser N. Factors influencing fatty acids in meat and the role of antioxidants in improving meat quality. *Br J Nutr* 1997;78(Suppl 1):S49-S60.
14. Siscovick DS, Raghunathan TE, et al. Dietary intake and cell membrane levels of long-chain n-3 polyunsaturated fatty acids and the risk of primary cardiac arrest." *JAMA* 1995;274(17):1363-1367.
15. Simopolous AP, Robinson J. The Omega Diet. HarperCollins; New York, 1999.
16. Rose DP, Connolly JM, et al. Influence of diets containing esapentaenoic or docasahexaenoic acid on growth and metastasis of breast cancer cells in nude mice. *J Natl Cancer Inst* 1995;87(8):587-592.
17. Tisdale MJ. Wasting in cancer. *J Nutr* 1999;129(1S Suppl):243S-246S.
18. Tashiro T, Yamamori H, et al. N-3 versus n-6 polyunsaturated fatty acids in critical illness. *Nutrition* 1998;14(6):551-553.
19. Russell JB, Diez-Gonzalez F, Jarvis GN. Potential effect of cattle diets on the transmission of pathogenic Escherichia coli to humans. *Microbes Infect* 2000;2(1):45-53.
20. Wood JD, Enser M, Fisher AV, et al. Manipulating meat quality and composition. *Proc Nutr Soc* 1999;58(2):363-370.
21. Mandell IB, Buchanan-Smith JP, Campbell CP. Effects of forage vs grain feeding on carcass characteristics, fatty acid composition, and beef quality in Limousin-cross steers when time on feed is controlled. *J Anim Sci* 1998;76(10):2619-2630.
22. Stunkard AJ, Wadden TA. (Editors) *Obesity: Theory and Therapy,* Second Edition. Raven Press; New York, 1993.
23. National Institutes of Health. *Clinical guidelines on the identification, evaluation, and treatment of overweight and obesity in adults.* Department of Health and Human Services, National Institutes of Health, National Heart, Lung, and Blood Institute;

Bethesda, Maryland, 1998.
24. Murray RK, Granner DK, Mayes PA, Rodwell VW. *Harper's Biochemistry.* Appleton & Lange; Stamford, Ct., 2000.
25. Classen B, Witthohn K, Blaschek W., Characterization of an arabinogalactan-protein isolated from pressed juice of *Echinacea purpurea* by precipitation with the beta-glucosyl Yariv reagent. *Carbohydr Res* 2000;327(4):497-504.
26. Zhang J, Wang G, Li H, et al. Antitumor polysaccharides from a Chinese mush-room, "yuhuangmo," the fruiting body of *Pleurotus citrinopileatus. Biosci Biotech Biochem* 1994;58(7):1195-1201.
27. Banerjee PC, Ghosh AK, Sengupta S. Hemagglutinating activity in extracts of mycelia from submerged mushroom cultures. *Appl Environ Microbiol* 1982;44(4): 1009-1011.
28. Jennemann R, Geyer R, Sandhoff R, et al. Glycoinositol phosphosphingolipids (basidiolipids) of higher mushrooms. *Eur J Biochem.* 2001;268(5):1190-1205.
29. Jennemann R, Bauer BL Bertalanffy H, et al. Novel glycoinositolphosphosphin-golipids, basidiolipids, from Agaricus. *Eur. J. Biochem.* 1999;259, 331-338.
30. Hirazumi A, Furusawa E. An immunomodulatory polysaccharide-rich substance from the fruit juice of Morinda citrifolia (noni) with antitumour activity. *Phytother Res.* 1999;13(5):380-387.
31. Furusawa E, Hirazumi A, Story S, Jensen J. Antitumour potential of a polysaccharide-rich substance from the fruit juice of Morinda citrifolia (noni) on sarcoma 180 ascites tumour in mice. *Phytother Res.* 2003;17(10):1158-1164.
32. Shils ME. *Modern Nutrition in Health and Disease,* 8th Edition. Lea & Febiger; Philadelphia, Pa., 1994.
33. Ramberg J, McAnalley BH. Is saccharide supplementation necessary? *GlycoScience & Nutrition.* 2002;3(3):1-9.
34. Cao G, Good SL, Sadowski JA, Prior RL. Increases in human plasma antioxidant capacity after consumption of controlled diets high in fruit and vegetables. *Am J Clin Nutr.* 1998;68:1081-1087.
35. Freeze HH. Disorders in protein glycosylation and potential therapy: Tip of an ice-berg? *J Pediatrics.* 1998;133(5):593-600.
36. Martin A, Rambal C, Berger V, et al. Availability of specific sugars for glycoconjugate biosynthesis: A need for further investigations in man. *Biochimie.* 1998;80 (1):75-86.
37. Alton G, Hasilik M, Niehues R. Direct utilization of mannose for mammalian glyco-protein biosynthesis. *Glycobiology.* 1998;8:285-295.
38. Axford JS. Glycosylation and rheumatic disease. *Proceedings of the Royal Society of Medicine's 5th Jenner Symposium (Glycobiology and Medicine conference),* July 10-11, 2000.
39. Axford J. Glycobiology & Medicine A Millennial Review. *GlycoScience & Nutrition* 2001;2(7).
40. Online Mendelian Inheritance in Man, OMIM™. McKusick-Nathans Institute for Genetic Medicine, Johns Hopkins University (Baltimore, MD) and National Center for Biotechnology Information, National Library of Medicine (Bethesda, MD), 2000: http://www.ncbi.nlm.nih.gov/omim/.
41. Lefkowitz DL. Glyconutritionals: implications in asthma. *GlycoScience & Nutrition.* 2000;1(15):1-4.
42. Gardiner T. Dietary fucose: absorption, distribution, metabolism, excretion (ADME) and biological activity. *GlycoScience & Nutrition.* 2000; 1(6):1-4.
43. Gardiner T. Dietary N-acetylneuraminic acid (NANA): absorption, distribution,

metabolism, excretion (ADME) and biological activity. *GlycoScience & Nutrition.* 2000; 1(10):1-3.

44. Lefkowitz SS. Glyconutritionals: implications for cancer. *GlycoScience & Nutrition.* 2000;1(14):1-3.

45. Lefkowitz DL. Glyconutritionals: implications in inflammation. *GlycoScience & Nutrition.* 2000;1(17):1-4.

46. Gauntt CJ, McAnalley BH, McDaniel HR. Glyconutritonals: implications for recovery from viral infections. *GlycoScience & Nutrition.* 2001;2(2):1-6.

47. Friedman MJ. Control of malaria virulence by alpha 1-acid glycoprotein (orosomucoid), an acute-phase (inflammatory) reactant. *Proc Natl Acad Sci USA.* 1983;80 (17):5421-5424.

48. Barragan A. A Spoonful of Sugar to Combat Malaria? *SCOPE Forum*, Washington University, December 14, 1999. http://scope.educ.washington.edu/malaria/update/show.php?author=Barragan&date=1999-12-14

49. Dykman KD, Ford CR, Tone CM. The effects of dietary supplements on lupus: a retrospective survey. *Proc Fisher Inst Med Res.* 1997;1:26-30.

50. Dykman KD, Ford CR, Horn E. Gardiner T. Effects of long-term nutritional supplementation on functionality in patients diagnosed with fibromyalgia and chronic fatigue syndrome. Poster Presentation at the American Association of Chronic Fatigue Syndrome 5th International Conference, January 26-29, 2001.

51. Dykman KD, Gardiner T, Ford CR, Horn E. The effects of long-term supplementation on the functionality and use of non-drug therapies in patients diagnosed with fibromyalgia and chronic fatigue syndrome. Poster Ppresentation at the Experimental Biology Annual Meeting, March 31-April 4, 2001.

52. Hyland G, Miller D. A pilot survey: standard cancer therapy combined with nutraceutical dietary supplementation improves treatment responses and patient quality of life. Oral Presentation: Comprehensive Cancer Care II: Integrating Complementary & Alternative Therapies. Crystal City, Arlington, VA; June, 1999.

53. Hall J, Boyd S. Case report: improved tolerance of cancer therapy in a patient taking glyconutritional supplementation. *GlycoScience & Nutrition.* 2002;3(2):1-4.

54. Ramberg J. How soon should I expect to experience the effects of dietary supplements? *GlycoScience & Nutrition.* 2001;2(1):1-2.

55. Barhoumi R, Burghardt RG, Busbee DL, et al. Enhancement of glutathione levels and protection from chemically initiated glutathione depletion in rat liver cells by glyconutritionals. *Proc Fisher Inst Med Res.* 197;1(1):12-16.

56. Busbee D, Barhoumi R, Burghardt RC, et al. Protection from glutathione depletion by a glyconutritional mixture of saccharides. *Age.* 1999;22(4):159-165.

57. Gardiner T. Pharmacokinetics and safety of glyconutritional sugars for use as dietary supplements. 2004;5(2):1-6.

58. Gardiner T, McAnalley BH, Vennum EP. Glyconutritionals: consolidated review of potential benefits from the scientific literature. *GlycoScience & Nutrition.* 2001;2 (15):1-17.

Additional Reading

1. Davidson MH, Hunninghake D, et al. Comparison of the effects of lean red meat vs lean white meat on serum lipid levels among free-living persons with hypercholesterolemia: a long-term, randomized clinical trial. *Arch Intern Med* 1999;159(12):1331-1338.

2. French P, Stanton C, Lawless F, et al. Fatty acid composition, including conjugated linoleic acid, of intramuscular fat from steers offered grazed grass, grass silage, or

concentrate-based diets. *J Anim Sci* 2000;78(11):2849-2855.

3. Duckett SK, Wagner DG, et al. Effects of time on feed on beef nutrient composition. *J Anim Sci* 1993;71(8): 2079-88.

4. Lopez-Bote CJ, Sanz Arias R, Rey AI, et al. Effect of free-range feeding on omega-3 fatty acids and alpha-tocopherol content and oxidative stability of eggs. *An Feed Sci Technol* 1998;72: 33-40.

5. Dolecek TA, Grandits G. Dietary polyunsaturated Ffty acids and mortality in the multiple risk factor intervention trial (MRFIT). *World Rev Nutr Diet* 1991;66:205-216.

6. Dhiman TR, Anand GR, et al. Conjugated linoleic acid content of milk from cows fed different diets. *J Dairy Sci* 1999; 82(10):2146-2156.

7. Ip C, Scimeca JA, et al. Conjugated linoleic acid. A powerful anti-carcinogen from animal fat sources. *Cancer* 1994;74(3 suppl):1050-1054.

8. Aro A, Mannisto S, Salminen I, et al. Inverse association between dietary and serum conjugated linoleic acid and risk of breast cancer in postmenopausal women. *Nutr Cancer* 2000;38(2):151-157.

9. Smith GC. Dietary supplementation of vitamin E to cattle to improve shelf life and case life of beef for domestic and international markets. *J Animal Sci* 1993;71(8): 2079-2088.

10. Allen VG, Fontenot JP, Kelly RF, Notter DR. Forage systems for beef production from conception to slaughter: III. Finishing systems. *J Anim Sci* 1996;74(3):625-638.

Chapter 10
Antioxidants–Your First Line of Defense

Much of this book has discussed threats to your health from environmental toxins. Toxins cause free radical activity in your body that can also be described as oxidative stress. Free radicals are a normal by-product of energy production, and the body is designed to cope with this natural process. But we now live in a world that has countless thousands of toxins that cause excessive free radicals to attack virtually every cell of your body. We are simply not designed to deal with that level of oxidative stress. The result is cell damage and disease.

Oxidative Stress–the most serious threat!
Oxidative stress can be understood by thinking of it as common rust. Rust is oxidative stress on metal. A similar process takes place on your cells. Free radicals attacking the integrity of the metal molecules cause it to decay and rot away. In fact, I recall when I was just a young teen trying to keep my old used car from falling apart. My friends and I used to refer to the rusting bodies of cars as having cancer. It's not far from what happens in your cells when free radicals attack them.

Free radicals, unchecked, <u>are</u> the principal cause of cancers. They are also the principal cause of heart diseases, as well as many other illnesses. Researchers have found that oxidative free radicals contribute to Alzheimer's disease, Parkinson's disease, diabetes, cataracts, arthritis and virtually all of the diseases and ailments associated with aging because the principal cause of aging is free radical oxidative stress.[1-3]

Yes, even some diseases previously thought to be strictly inherited like Parkinson's disease may actually be caused by or at least worsened by free radicals caused by toxins in our environment. In the case of Parkinson's, farm pesticides are the primary suspects. Why? Because certain chemical toxins affect the nervous system, but there are those that are known to damage human DNA, and that certainly could affect our genetic makeup.

There is an increasing body of data supporting the idea that environmental toxins at least contribute to (and may even cause) ADD, ADHD and other cognitive disorders. Although there is valid research to show that numerous factors exacerbate the symptoms of ADD and ADHD in all age groups, the strong possibility that neurotoxic agents in the environment may contribute to the incidence of this behavior needs to be seriously considered. Studies must be conducted on the effects of specific toxins, such as PCBs and lead, both in adults and children. Research indicates that ADHD patients who are individually managed with supplementation, dietary modification, detoxification, correction of intestinal dysbiosis (commonly, although not always correctly, referred to by laymen as candida), and other features of a holistic/integrative program of management can lead normal, productive lives without pharmaceuticals.[4-7]

As we examine the evidence on oxidative stress in this book, it will become clear that, for the majority of health issues today, a holistic or complementary approach keyed on antioxidants and diet modification are essential if you wish to enjoy true wellness.

Antioxidants may be helpful with other inflammatory issues, fatigue and mental acuity.[8-17] In addition, they act as important protection for your skin against the ravages of free radicals and damaging ultraviolet radiation from the sun.[18] We have some very interesting data on antioxidants and inflammation as well as fatigue, and when you understand antioxidants, information like this just makes sense.

A Nutritional Cocktail for the Brain?

Degeneration of brain cells over time leading to cognitive dysfunction (such as in Alzheimer's and related dementias) is a growing concern, But I believe that there is more hope in this area than most people imagine. According to research published in a journal called *Clinical Geriatric Medicine,* in addition to pharmaceuticals such as statins and antihypertensive agents that ameliorate the effects of even genetically induced cognitive dysfunction, antioxidants and estrogen replacement can positively affect age-related factors. By altering the balance between neuronal injury and repair, we can delay the expression and progression of the neurodegenerative processes of brain aging, Alzheimer's and related dementias.[14]

Along with the recommendations I have made for years regarding brain function–and, in fact, most of the nutritional "cocktail" I made for my son when he miraculously survived viral encephalitis–antioxidants alone have been shown in clinical study to delay many neuronal effects of aging and to restore normal memory for a variety of tasks.[15] Antioxidants help neutralize tissue-damaging free radicals, which become more prevalent as organisms age. It is hypothesized that increasing antioxidant levels in an organism might retard or reverse the damaging effects of free radicals on neurons.[15]

I'll discuss my son's case further in a later chapter, but I'm sure that right now you're eager to know what was in his nutritional cocktail. The contents included phosphatidylserine (PS), phosphatidylcholine (PC), L-carnitine (ALC) and antioxidants, particularly vitamin E and quercetin, plus ginkgo biloba. Of course, I also added a balance of vitamins and both macro- and microminerals. That saved his brain function but did not stop the epileptic seizures. To learn how things turned out, you'll just have to continue reading!

I have frequently discussed (and will do so again!) diet modifications, as well as lifestyle changes and supplementation. One very interesting study from Tufts University examined the possibility of slowing age-related cognitive degeneration with a sharp increase in antioxidants from fruit or vegetable extracts. The researchers found that antioxidants did indeed retard this process. In fact, the study told us, "Nutritional interventions–in this case, increasing dietary intake of fruits and vegetables–can retard and even reverse age-related declines in brain function and in cognitive and motor performance in rats. Our lab has shown that as Fischer 344 rats age, their brains are increasingly vulnerable to oxidative stress. *Dietary supplementation with fruit or vegetable extracts high in antioxidants can decrease this vulnerability to oxidative stress.*"[16]

Do these lab results indicate that we can slow or perhaps even reverse the age-related degeneration of the human brain with antioxidants? I believe we can, but until an irrefutable study is done to prove that, I must reiterate that antioxidants are necessary in higher levels in food than previously thought–far higher, in fact, than most people will eat. Bearing this fact in mind, food supplementation becomes the logical choice. If used correctly, supplements can't harm you, so what do you have to lose by trying? According to scientific study, even if you take only vitamin E–far from the best antioxidant supplement available–you can reduce the effects of cognitive dysfunction related to aging.[17]

As discussed earlier, glyconutrients are vital for every major function. But they cannot protect you from the level of oxidative stress we have today without additional, very potent antioxidant support. When I say "potent," I do not mean mega-

dosing; I mean the most efficient antioxidants combined in the most synergistic way. A small number of milligrams combined correctly can yield more effective results than mega-doses of single or poorly combined antioxidants.[19,20] Without question, antioxidants are the single, most important defense for your body in our current, 21st-century world.

What you need for complete antioxidant protection
1. Vitamins that are antioxidants
   - Vitamins A, C and E
2. Mineral synergists to antioxidants
   - Selenium and zinc
3. Phytochemicals
   - Flavonoids, indoles, etc.
4. Glyconutrients
   - For the production and protection of glutathione

Synergistic Partners in Health

Nutritional biochemistry is far more complex than most people (including most doctors) may realize. As I frequently say, nutritional biochemistry is a giant, connect-the-dots game that involves all nutrient groups, co-factors and enzymes. All too frequently, the drug mentality that dominates Western society leads patients and doctors to think that, if they have a particular primary factor such as vitamin A, then everything else will automatically function correctly. This false but pervasive belief is one of the reasons that doctors are given such limited training to recognize health issues as they relate to dietary deficiencies and why tests available to them from medical labs are also very limited.

Some antioxidant vitamins are well-known, such as A, C and E. However, there are also minerals that are synergistic to antioxidant vitamins. Less well-known is that vitamins and minerals are partners so to speak; and, if you wish certain vitamins to function optimally, their synergistic partner needs to be present. The presence of a synergist (some would say a "catalyst") is just as important as the primary antioxidant. For example, selenium is the synergist for vitamin E. If you supplement by taking vitamin E but are selenium-deficient, you will not get the full benefits of vitamin E. Selenium is also essential to immune, heart and thyroid function.[21-23]

All glands require multiple nutritional support. Since thyroid dysfunction is probably the best-known problem in the eyes of the public, I'll give you an example of synergy involving that gland. If your thyroid is to function correctly, it also needs at a minimum the minerals iodine, selenium, manganese and magnesium. Selenium may be more important to healthy thyroid than previously believed. If someone with thyroid disorder has both selenium and iodine deficiencies at the same time, adverse reactions will be magnified. Selenium levels may therefore have major influence on the outcome of iodine deficiency in both human and animal populations.[21,22]

Both selenium and magnesium need vitamin B6 in order to function correctly, and the thyroid requires a minimum of one amino acid–tyrosine.[24] Just connect the dots. If you neglect any synergist or catalyst your body needs, you experience dysfunction, and dysfunction leads to disease. It really is just that simple.

Zinc and vitamins C and A all have specialized functions. They are particularly important partners for immune function, and all must be present in order to ensure complete immune function and antioxidant support. With this knowledge in mind, be sure you take a multiple vitamin and mineral supplement daily, along with your antioxidant supplement.

I believe this book makes it clear that you cannot be 100% certain you are getting enough of any nutrient these days. To show how complex and complicated nutritional biochemistry is, zinc won't function without B_6, nor can some enzymes be made without it.[25,26] Every nutrient requires other nutrients as co-factors, either for activation or function from each of the nutrient categories, vitamins, minerals and amino acids. No nutrient is an island unto itself. For activation, all of the nutrients mentioned above require enzymes, and for function, essential fatty acids (EFAs) are also needed.[27,28]

People taking EFA supplements who are deficient in EFA co-factors are generally doing no more than producing expensive urine. According to research on EFAs done by a Dr. Das, "Micronutrients, vitamins A, C, and E, beta-carotene and selenium can decrease the incidence of cancer, possibly due to their antioxidant action(s). These nutrients prevent lipid peroxidation, especially that of gamma-linolenic (GLA), dihomo-gamma-linolenic (DGLA) and arachidonic acids (AA), which are the precursors of prostaglandins.[28]

Prostaglandins (PGs) are substances that are often mistakenly identified as hormones. They do closely resemble hormones in some ways. However PGs are actually the carbon-20 unsaturated fatty acids that are found in all mammals. They provide a number of functions, including the control of smooth muscle contraction, blood pressure, inflammation and body temperature. Are EFAs important? It would seem so, but there are even more facts available.

Dr. Das continued by saying that, "Gamma-linolenic acid (GLA), dihomo-gamma-linolenic acid (DGLA), prostaglandin E1 (PGE1) and prostacyclin can prevent genetic damage *in vitro* and *in vivo*." These work together to augment immune responses and tumoricidal actions of macrophages. In plain language, don't expect your immune cells that are called macrophages, which is Latin for big eater, to eat tumor cells without the proper EFA support. Prostacyclin also has anti-metastatic properties. Zinc, magnesium, calcium and pyridoxine (B_6) are co-factors in the formation of GLA, DGLA, PGE1 and PGI2. Hence, in situations where there is reduced intake of trace elements and vitamins, there may also be a decrease in the synthesis of GLA, DGLA, PGE1 and PGI2, leading to immune suppression and genetic damage that cannot be reversed or prevented."[28] This interaction between nutrients, essential fatty acids and prostaglandins can be exploited to develop new preventive and therapeutic strategies in cancer. So in plain language, be sure you are taking a multivitamin/mineral and EFA supplement if you want to have the best chance of success in cancer.

Even the Best Is Not Enough

Now let's make this equation even more complex:

We know that we should eat fresh and raw fruits and vegetables because that is what we are designed to do. We also know that processing of any type causes food to lose nutritional value. *However even if you buy the best raw fresh fruits and vegetables, what you get nutritionally will vary from one item to another.* Even two fruits from the same tree will vary in nutritional content. Different plant species containing the same vitamin, for example, will vary in content of that vitamin. For example, the vitamin C content of a grape, an orange and broccoli are different. Soil mineral conditions, the growing season, time of harvest, and the use of herbicides or plant regulators all affect the nutrient content of many fresh foods.[29-31]

Nutritional content of food also varies not only with the source, but also with what the source was fed. One example of this is the levels of vitamin A, vitamin D, vitamin E and carotenoids in milk. Nutritional intake increases if a cow feeds on green grass, as opposed to hay.[32] That makes sense, doesn't it? After all, cows were designed to eat grass, not hay and certainly not corn meal.

There is a highly contested concept of vine-ripened vs. green harvest and gassing to artificially make fruit appear to have actually ripened naturally. The scientific facts are clear in this matter–despite what the commercial grocery industry would have you believe. Carotenoid levels generally increase in fruits as they naturally ripen.[33] That would be reason enough, but there is more.

Tomatoes, well-known for their healthful lycopene content, have higher levels of that micronutrient if they are given time to vine-ripen. They also have higher beta-carotene and soluble fiber than tomatoes ripened off the vine under otherwise identical environmental conditions.[34]

If you are not convinced yet, let's make our case even stronger: At least two recent studies reported that our fresh fruits and vegetables are lower in certain vitamins and minerals today than they were as recently as 30 years ago. One analysis compared levels of seven vitamins and minerals found in 25 common fruits and vegetables between 1951 and 1999. The overall nutrient losses far exceeded the nutrient gains.[35]

Hard-working, intelligent people who study to become dietitians are not being taught this crucial data. Neither are doctors. They do not learn, for example, that losses of vital nutrients from foods are far greater than they could imagine.

Some of those foods and their nutrients include broccoli (calcium, riboflavin, vitamin A and vitamin C), spinach (riboflavin and vitamin E), and potatoes, cauliflower, strawberries, tomatoes and green peppers (vitamin C).[35]

Here is one more surprise. One serving of broccoli would have supplied more than the current RDA of vitamin A for adult males in 1951. Today you would have to eat more than two servings to obtain the same amount of vitamin A. Two peaches would have supplied the current RDA of vitamin A for adult women in 1951. Today, a woman would have to eat almost 53 peaches to meet her daily requirements! That's right–53 of today's peaches to equal the nutrition from one peach grown in 1951.[35] No, I didn't make a mistake: I don't mean vitamin C. I know peaches have more C than A, but I am trying to make a point with the data from this study.

Another study compared data collected in 1930 and 1980 for eight minerals in 40 fruits and vegetables. The study's author reported significant losses of calcium, magnesium, copper and sodium in vegetables, and magnesium, iron, copper and potassium in fruits. These foods were also significantly higher in water and lower in fiber content.[36]

Why Nutrient Loss Occurs
Why do these nutrient losses happen? The author of the above study cited numerous possible factors, including current methods of plant breeding that select for post-harvest handling qualities and cosmetic appeal rather than nutrient content. Also playing a role in nutrient loss were changed storage and ripening systems and greater reliance on chemical fertilizers, both of which have contributed to soil nutrient losses.

Few people think about loss of nutrition due to storage methods. There have been some interesting findings in this area. The short list below just scratches the surface. For more details read a paper called "From the Farm to the Kitchen Table: A Review of the Nutrient Losses in Foods" by Jane Ramberg and Bill McAnalley.[37]

Most stored fresh vegetables steadily lose vitamin C.[36] For example, green beans refrigerated after harvest lost more than 90% of their vitamin C after 16 days of refrigeration. Broccoli lost about 50% of both vitamin C and beta-carotene after five days of storage.[38]

Following cold storage for eight days in the light, spinach lost 22% of lutein content. In eight days of dark cold, spinach lost 18% of its beta-carotene. On the bright side, however, carrot carotenoids remained stable under both conditions.[39] We also find significant losses of vitamin C in orange juice that is stored in polyethylene or wax paper containers. Vitamin retention is better in glass containers.[29]

Another piece of interesting evidence can be found in the table below:

A researcher named Souci (previously mentioned) did some truly excellent work on the analysis of nutritional content of vitamins, minerals, saccharides, antioxidants and phytohormones from fruits and vegetables. Ramberg and McAnalley used Souci's data to compare the actual loss of these nutrients from fresh raw foods following various heat processing methods.[37] They found that the information posted by the United States Department of Agriculture (USDA) is very far from accurate. But that is the information used by dietitians, doctors and university nutrition science departments. Just take a look at the huge discrepancies between what the so-called experts believe will be lost in food processing and the shocking reality of what will actually happen:

Table 1
Nutrient losses when fruits and vegetables are canned: A Comparison of USDA Nutrient Retention Factors (estimates) vs. Actual Nutrient Analysis USDA's Table from[37]

Nutrient	Percent loss estimates	Percent loss calculated
calcium	5%	28%
magnesium	0%	34%
zinc	0%	53%
vitamin C	50%	76%
thiamine	20%	83%
riboflavin	10%	50%
niacin	10%	40%
vitamin B6	0%	34%
folate	50%	71%
vitamin A (retinol equivalents)	0%	34%
carotenoids	25%	42%

•canned fruit
**canned fruits and vegetables

The above table shows the amount of vitamin C in raw, boiled and canned fruits and vegetables. Heat, to any extent, will reduce nutritional content of the food. In today's world, attempting to reach the RDA (required daily allowance) is not sufficient. The required daily amount, regardless of what it's called in different countries, is simply the minimum nutrition necessary to keep from becoming a victim of nutritional deficiency disease over time. It is not–I repeat, *not*–the maximum that you can take before you become toxic from a dietary supplement.

Of course, vitamin/mineral supplementation varies from person to person. Governments try to give a reasonable, safe, average minimum based on whatever they believe to be accurate data. Sometimes that data is accurate and, as you have learned in this book, sometimes it isn't. Therefore, it is entirely possible that the government information in any specific country regarding the daily requirement may be based on out-of-date or inaccurate data. I wish I had the staff and the time to verify the data for each nation, but I don't. Still, there are studies offered in this book that show a definite need to update data in many countries with regard to certain nutrients that have been studied.

Available foods and the varying content of certain minerals in the soil also influence the minimum daily amount set in each country. Some areas of the world have higher levels of copper in their food, or even copper in the dust that people breathe. In these areas, copper supplementation is not advisable.

In other regions, levels of copper or iron may be too high. So multiple vitamin/mineral products should be copper- or iron-free for people in those places. Copper, iron and zinc compete with each other. So it would be possible to have a health issue such as iron anemia result from having excessive amounts of zinc or copper, for example. Back to the old connect-the-dots game again.

When I was in practice, I would test my patients for iron, copper and zinc to determine if they would benefit from having a special supplement void of iron or copper. Those who were taking excess zinc for immune function or prostate problems got a serious talking to from me. I limited the amount of zinc they were allowed to take. I found most of my patients were better off with an iron-free, multiple vitamin supplement, the most notable exception being vegetarian patients, who very often would benefit from extra iron. There were, however, a few vegetarians educated well enough who did not need that supplementation.

Iron, copper and zinc are called macrominerals. They are required in milligram (mg) levels. Trace minerals, however, are called microminerals and are required in only microgram (mcg) levels. Micro- or trace minerals are essential for direct antioxidant activity in addition to functioning as co-factors for a variety of antioxidant enzymes.

Interestingly, many doctors do not realize the importance of trace minerals in maintaining optimal health. They would no doubt be surprised to learn of trace elements' significance in wound healing and immune function, for example. A deficiency state can develop very quickly in critically ill patients due to decreased nutrient intakes and, more importantly, increased nutrient requirements. Daily intakes up to or exceeding many times the RDA usually are required under these conditions.[23,40] It would be exceedingly unwise to chance a deficiency in terms of prevention, but it is crucially important to ensure that deficiency states will not occur during an illness, or the healing process may be significantly impaired.

When Deficiencies Happen...

As much as a third of the world's population does not meet their physical and intellectual potential because of vitamin and mineral deficiencies, according to a report released by UNICEF and The Micronutrient Initiative.[41] **We typically assume that this is a problem only in developing nations, but it is happening worldwide. Generally,** most people can benefit from an increase in one or more trace minerals in their diets, but this kind of increase must be assessed on a case-by-case basis. Once again, being free of obvious symptoms does not indicate that all is well. Deficiency symptoms are usually very subtle–sometimes for extended periods of time–as one system robs another to try to keep you going.

As already mentioned, many governments are moving forward based on outdated human nutrition information. Sadly, they are not current on the threats mentioned in this book and, in most cases, never learn about the role of nutrients in disease prevention and healing. Nor do they learn that deficiencies often occur in specific nutrients (in addition to the more obvious ones) during the stress of an illness.

Soil depletion isn't just a result of over-farming–it is a preventable reality. Researchers are now concerned that dietary selenium (Se) intake is inadequate for the populations in the UK and parts of Europe.[23]

In Finland, soil deficiencies of selenium were recognized, and the method used to deal with this problem was the addition of selenium to fertilizer. That method will work, but only at an extra expense to the grower. In the U.S. and perhaps other countries, corporate farmers are unlikely to spend the money even if they recognize the problem, so the responsibility for paying once again falls on the consumer. Selenium (Se) is an essential component of at least twenty functional proteins within mammals. These proteins are essential for a range of metabolic functions, including thyroid hormone synthesis and immune functions, as I explained earlier. They are also vital for antioxidant activity, and increased Se intake has the potential to influence a very wide range of factors that may help lower the incidence of chronic diseases.[42]

In various countries, some trace minerals are still in good supply in the soil. *But that abundance will not last unless we go back to the proper soil rotation methods and begin to control population growth.* One of the few trace minerals still found in sufficient supply in some places is selenium, but in many cases these levels are only sufficient for an already healthy person to maintain their health. They are rarely sufficient to make a difference for patients already in a disease state. Also, too much selenium can also lead to serious health problems. Once again, I recommend case-by-case assessment. Only proper testing by a doctor trained in this area (not the average physician) can determine this need. Once again, I caution you not to self-prescribe or self-medicate.

The U.S. has long been referred to as the breadbasket of the world. But in our attempts to feed the world, we have depleted most of our soil through modern farming methods.

Soil across the U.S. is not always rich in selenium, and, depending on the specific individual, substantial levels of selenium supplementation (short-term) can be very beneficial. Not only would it be for heart and thyroid patients as mentioned above and as a synergist to vitamin E, but it is also essential for healthy prostate glands. The older a man is, the more likely he is to need to supplement his selenium level.

How Much is Too Much?

I have alluded to toxicity of certain nutrients, but I do not want you to have the wrong impression: Generally speaking, most minerals have to be at incredible levels before you reach toxicity. As an example, the toxic level of magnesium is 30,000mg per day. Since as little as 100 mg's daily of magnesium will loosen your stool (sometimes uncomfortably so) and the more you take the looser it gets, no one could ever take that much.

The likelihood of a deficiency is far greater than that of toxicity when it comes to vitamins and minerals. Some nutrients are water-soluble and some are fat-soluble. In most cases only the fat soluble ones present any possibility for concern. We'll cam back to them in a moment. It is nearly impossible to become toxic from the majority of vitamins that are water-soluble. It is also difficult in most cases to become toxic from most minerals by using most supplements daily. Mega-dosing of certain nutritional minerals such as iron, zinc, copper and selenium, however, can be very dangerous. I have for years recommended limits in these areas and have cautioned my patients to use restraint with those nutrients unless directed to go above the minimums by a health professional specifically trained in the therapeutic use of dietary supplements.

Iron Supplementation--Yea or Nay?

I have also counseled against the supplementation of iron for most people for many years. Although an essential mineral, iron may contribute to free radical activity and heart disease in some patients, as well as lowering their immune function.[43,44] The leading cause of poisoning in American children is the excess iron they get from children's chewable vitamins.[45,46] Having said that, there are parts of the world where iron is deficient, so once again proper testing before use is strongly recommended.

Since I have been frequently questioned for my recommendations against broad daily general iron supplementation and criticized for designing multiple vitamin and mineral products without iron this is a good place to tell you why I have done so. The issue of iron overload is more serious than even many doctors are aware of. Iron overload can be caused be genetic conditions that I will cover shortly but also by, accidental ingestion, repeated blood transfusions, **inhalation of tobacco smoke** (stay away from cigarette smoke!) or asbestos, over medication with iron supplements or iron pills prescribed by a physician and be present in certain types of anemia and porphyrias.

Ok now you want to know what porphyrias are. It's a disease of metabolism caused by the body's failure to metabolize porphyrins. Porphyrins are any of various organic compounds that are common in animal and plant tissue, for example, as components of hemoglobin, chlorophyll, and some enzymes. They consist of four pyrrole rings linked by methylene groups. Symptoms of the hereditary form of the disease include abdominal pain, sensitivity to sunlight, confusion, and excretion of porphyrins in the urine. Whether your interested or not I can't help myself I have a need to tell people about the root of words, call it a quirk. The word porphyrin is derived from the Greek porphura, which means purple. Ok probably a lot more than you wanted to know so let's get back to iron overload.

To add to the reasons **not** to have iron daily in a dietary supplement there is something called hereditary hemochromatosis (HH), also known as iron overload disease or "genetic iron poisoning". It is the most common genetic disease in the U.S.A. according to the U.S. Centers for Disease Control and Prevention (CDC) in Atlanta, Georgia. It is due to a mutation of a particular gene, *HFE*, that regulates iron absorption.

It is an active genetic disease in 1 out of every 250 people of European decent on average. Genetic iron overload may not be exclusive to Europeans or even to Caucasians in general however. It is now suspected that there is a different type of genetic iron overload that affects Africans called African siderosis. Additional studies are needed to confirm that a genetic defect may also be implicated in iron overload in Africans. Regardless hereditary hemochromatosis can occur in African Americans, although not nearly as frequently as in Caucasians.

In North America one in 8 are "silent carriers" of the single HH gene mutation and 1 in 100-200 have the double mutation putting them at high risk for developing full-blown HH. HH can affect men, women and children at any age. Most of the approximately 33 million Americans who have the HH gene mutation don't know it but your doctor can diagnose it easily and quickly with a simple blood draw.

Hemochromatosis is a disorder in which there is excess accumulation of iron in the body leading to damage of many organs, especially the liver and pancreas.

What are the symptoms of Hemochromatosis:
- Persistent Fatigue/Tiredness
- Abdominal discomfort
- Swollen liver
- Raised liver enzymes
- Fatty liver
- Joint pains
- Loss of sex drive
- Bronzed coloration to the skin (due to melanin deposition)
- The triad of bronze skin, enlarged liver and Diabetes mellitus is only present in cases of gross iron overload.

Not every one who suffers from HH will have all the symptoms nor do the symptoms necessarily have to be severe. If you have any of these symptoms it would be smart to check with your doctor and request that he or she perform the HFE gene analysis for C282Y mutation. This simply requires a blood sample.

Unlike many other nutrients, iron is still in abundant supply in animal products– particularly red meat–and the redder the meat, the higher the iron content. All animal products contain iron since it is the core of red blood. Vegetarians also get some iron in their diets, but, in most cases they get less per ounce of food they consume than those who follow an omnivorous diet.

Lastly of course is that fact that unnecessary iron in you blood stream contributes to free radical problems particularly to heart disease. Testing will easily show if you need iron or if you suffer from iron overload. Considering the negatives with iron supplementation I suggest you don't use a supplement with iron unless you know you need it for certain.

Everyone has probably heard of hemoglobin, which in simple terms is composed of a) heme, which is the deep red, non-protein portion of hemoglobin that contains iron and b) globin, which refers to the protein portion. Hemoglobin is the substance in blood that transports oxygen from the lungs to body tissues. In general terms, a red blood cell is called a hemocyte. The word hemo is derived from Latin, and cyte was originally derived from the Greek word *kutos* (meaning receptacle), so they are in fact iron receptacles. Without iron we would die, but with too much of it we will also die. **Wellness is balance, and balance means wellness. That is the real trick–achieving and maintaining healthy balance to cope with the extraordinary conditions of the 21st century.**

Accentuate the Positive Response
This book is not about vitamin/mineral supplementation. Space does not allow an in-

depth explanation of what type of people should take what types or amounts of vitamins or minerals. Suffice it to say that you must take a daily supplement that provides you with at least the required daily amount, depending on the country you live in, your state of health, your genetics and your levels of stress.

For example, some of you will understand that adding additional water-soluble vitamins like B_{12}, or various other water-soluble vitamins, will give you nothing but a positive response.

I'll deviate for a moment here to answer a popular question and shatter a persistent myth: Vitamin B_2 (riboflavin) will make your urine turn yellow, but it is not–I repeat, not–an indicator of general vitamin absorption or the lack of it. It is only an indicator of B_2 passing through your body–nothing more definite than that. Nor does it mean you did not absorb any B_2–it simply shows you already had more B_2 in your fluids that you could have used during that particular period of time. So it is not an indicator of a good or bad quality vitamin product, as so many are fond of saying. Flavones, flavonoids and all other nutrients with similar names are all yellowish or in the yellow to orange family.

Now that that's settled, let's get back to the idea of toxicity. Vitamins that are fat-soluble (including vitamins A and E, as discussed earlier in this chapter) can become toxic at extremely high levels. But these levels are typically far higher than one would expect. Vitamin D is fat-soluble, but it isn't an antioxidant.

Critics of nutritional therapies will state that studies of antioxidants are contradictory. But most of those same critics have an agenda and are picking and choosing to suit their agendas. They are not being objective. In most cases, scientific studies are narrowly focused and consider only one item, or phenomenon, at a time. Antioxidants work! It is a question of synergy, not mega-dosing or isolation of nutrients. We have to stop thinking of nutrients as medicines and start thinking of them as food.

Two studies involving health professionals showed a significant reduction in cardiovascular disease among those with the highest intake of vitamin E, with an optimal intake range being from 100 to 249 IU per day.[47,48] These doses are impossible to get from food and can only be achieved by people who take food supplements.[19] Interestingly, the NAS daily RDA of vitamin E is 14.9 IU for adult males and 11.92 IU for adult females daily.[49] There seems to be a very large discrepancy between minimum government requirements and optimal levels, at least according to these particular studies of vitamin E.[47,48]

Several other studies done with beta-carotene in isolation and in huge amounts did not yield positive results. Antioxidants do work, but those wanting to prove that antioxidants or any nutritional supplements were bad could do two things: First, they could isolate a pro-vitamin like beta-carotene, dooming the study to failure since pro-vitamins are precursors–not vitamins–and should never be used as a therapy in isolation. Second, they could study the antioxidant or nutrient at a mega-dose level, which should never be done.

Beta-Carotene–Pro and Con

The most frequently used studies cited by the pro-pharmaceutical, anti-vitamin crowd to argue against the use of antioxidant dietary supplements are specifically focused on beta-carotene.[19,50-52] Shortly you'll learn why using beta-carotene (or any single isolate from complex) as an indicator for antioxidant protection is not the best choice. Let's take a look at what these studies demonstrated:

In the alpha-tocopherol/beta-carotene trial (ATBC), they reviewed the effect of 50mg of one form of vitamin E (alpha-tocopherol) combined with 20mg of beta-carotene, or 20mg of beta-carotene alone, based on the incidence of lung cancer among male smokers over a period of from 5 to 8 years. Researchers found an increase in lung cancer in subjects who took beta-carotene alone. The study also failed to demonstrate a favorable interaction between alpha-tocopherol and beta-carotene in regard to the incidence of lung cancer.[50]

The beta-carotene/retinol efficacy trial (CARET) involved 18,314 subjects who were at high risk for developing lung cancer (former or current smokers and workers exposed to asbestos). Subjects were given 30mg of beta-carotene per day and 25,000 IU of vitamin A or a placebo. The study was terminated 21 months early because the rate of cancer among those taking supplements was 28% higher than those taking the placebo. The rate of death from heart disease was 17% higher for those who took supplements.[51]

The Physicians' Health Study lasted 13 years and involved 22,071 male physicians assigned to take either 50mg of beta-carotene on alternate days or a placebo. Researchers found no appreciable difference between the placebo group and the group taking beta-carotene concerning the incidence of malignant neoplasms, cardiovascular disease or death from any other cause. The results suggest that long-term supplementation with beta-carotene provides no benefit at all.[52]

In another study that lasted 4 years, patients receiving 25mg of beta-carotene daily showed no reduction in the formation of colorectal cancer. The same study also failed to find preventive effects of daily doses of vitamin C or 400mg of vitamin E in respect to the development of colorectal cancer.[53]

A number of hypotheses have been postulated to explain the destructive effects of beta-carotene supplementation. Some hold that the doses used were too high, and others provide evidence that, in high oxygen concentrations and at high doses, beta-carotene was a weak pro-oxidant.[54,55]

An *in vitro* study by Palozza et al. demonstrated the effect of dose on beta-carotene behavior. At low concentrations (i.e. less than or equal to 25µM), they found that beta-carotene performed weakly as an antioxidant. However, at concentrations between 50 and 100µM, beta-carotene significantly acted as a pro-oxidant, increasing the production of ROS (reactive oxygen species, another way of saying harmful free radicals).[56] Several other studies have noted that beta-carotene behaves as a pro-oxidant under high oxygen partial pressures.[54,55,57]

Due to the high level of oxygen in the lungs' tissues, it follows that beta-carotene supplementation should promote the formation of, or exacerbate, pre-existing lung cancer.[55,57]

Prior to these studies, beta-carotene had been acknowledged as an antioxidant pro-vitamin. Indeed, beta-carotene, as it occurs naturally in food such as carrots, does offer some antioxidant benefit if consumed as a food. A pro-vitamin is a vitamin precursor, meaning that it is a substance that is converted into an active vitamin as a result of the body's normal biochemical processes. In the case of beta-carotene, it becomes vitamin A. Vitamin A is one the most important antioxidants. According to Koepke et al, factors such as air quality and composition (oxygen content), smoking, drinking alcohol, exercise and diet may have affected the results of those studies listed above. Researchers have identified other variables that also affect the behavior of antioxidants. Unbound metal ions, the amount of oxygen, the number of radicals, and the presence of co-antioxidants in a system, as well as dosage, can influence whether a compound behaves as an antioxidant or a pro-oxidant.[19]

What does that mean in plain language? In order to make a firm decision about whether beta-carotene or any other nutrient is healthful, all the above-mentioned factors must be considered. Beta-carotene was never meant to be mega-dosed or isolated from its co-factors. That makes it a medicine, not a nutrient. Testing for beta-carotene alone may give you useful preliminary information but is simply not a good indicator of the total antioxidant protection in your blood. In fact, according to the studies just mentioned, it may indicate something very negative in some people under certain conditions.

What one group of scientists discovered, after nearly four years of studies concluded in 2003, is that some proven individual antioxidants, given in high doses, cause a neutralizing or even a pro-oxidative effect. They also found that some antioxidants, when given separately from their synergistic co-factors, could also have a neutralizing or even harmful (pro-oxidative) effect. Pro-oxidative means that it contributes to free radical disease in the body. *Studies done from 2000 to 2003 indicated that synergy is the key to antioxidant effectiveness–not isolation or mega-dosing.*[19,58]

Feel the Phyto-Power!

Let's look at other antioxidant factors besides vitamins and minerals. You also need antioxidants from flavonoids such as quercetin in your daily diet. These are co-factors or synergists for antioxidant activity. Flavonoids belong to a bigger group called phytochemicals.

The word *phyto* is originally from the Greek word *phuton*, meaning plant. It was later modified in Latin to phyto. So whenever you see phyto as a prefix, it has something to do with a plant. The chemicals from the plant are then called phytochemicals. Many phytochemicals actually nourish the body or support a healthy function. These are called phytonutrients. Phytonutrients are not vitamins, minerals or herbals, but rather are specific chemicals found to occur naturally in plants. Phytonutrients are healthful to you, but cannot replace vitamins or minerals. Phytochemicals, such as flavonoids and indoles, function as antioxidants and free radical scavengers to protect plants from highly reactive oxygen radicals, sunlight, weather and viruses. (I will discuss flavonoids in greater detail later.)

Humans are designed to benefit from eating plants that contain disease-fighting phytochemicals. They are abundant in cruciferous vegetables like broccoli, brussels sprout, cabbage, cauliflower, kale and turnip. You know–the stuff most parents can't get their kids to eat! Phytonutrients are found in smaller levels in many other vegetables and fruits as well.[58] That is the reason those vegetables are so highly recommended in our diet and serve as the basis for some nutritional supplements. Some phytochemicals also help detoxify your body.

If everyone ate ten servings of raw fruits and vegetables daily, it would benefit our bodies significantly. But it would be extremely rare to find anyone who does that.

There are also antioxidants produced by your body such as glutathione and super oxide dismutase better known as SOD.

We have previously discussed glyconutrients. Among their many benefits is one that has been scientifically validated by a study involving scientists from two universities–

University of Texas and Texas A&M. They found that the glyconutrient complex actually raised glutathione *in vitro*. In fact, the glyconutrient complex raised glutathione levels in healthy cells by 20% and protected against depletion of glutathione by 50% when the cells were subjected to direct toxic chemical assault.[59] That result is very impressive and was totally unexpected since glyconutrients test zero as antioxidants on the standard method for testing antioxidants, which I will explain shortly.

The toxin used in the study is called patchulin, which is a mycotoxin. The study shows a significant benefit in adding glyconutrients, even when subjected to toxic chemical assault. According to Dr. Les Packer at the University of California at Berkeley, a leading expert in antioxidants, you cannot eat enough food to get sufficient glutathione in today's environment to protect you from free radical stress.[60]

If you cannot eat enough food to accomplish this health goal, you need it to protect your body from oxidative stress and cleanse your body, and the only sensible thing to do is to take a dietary supplement that can raise your glutathione levels in plasma. One of every three Americans will get cancer. That percentage is approximately the same for most modern nations. Experts estimate that 30-40% of the cancer cases are caused directly by poor diet.[61] I think I have already presented ample evidence on dietary stress in this book to convince any reasonable person that food alone simply cannot protect you from today's numerous stress factors.

Of course the main idea that inspired this book is toxins that cause health risks, premature aging and even death. One of those categories of toxins is labeled as carcinogenic (cancer-causing) agents. It's very simple: If your exposure to carcinogenic agents is increased, you increase the risk and often the occurrence of cancers. Decrease those agents in the environment and lower the risk of cancer. Increasing antioxidants to optimal (not mega) levels can also decrease your risk of cancer and other free radical related health issues.

Interim Measures

Even if all the world's leaders jumped on the environmental bandwagon today, we could not correct our toxic environment very quickly, so we have to do something for ourselves in the interim. That means modifying our diets in accordance with what is presented in this book, changing our lifestyles to avoid known oxidative stress agents as pointed out here, and taking antioxidant nutrients. Antioxidants lower cancer risk by neutralizing the free radicals that initiate cancer and other degenerative disease, as well as help to slow the aging process. We simply don't consume enough antioxidant in our daily diets to cope with today's free radical stress.

One leading expert in antioxidant research, Dr. Bruce Ames, estimates the average person takes about 10,000 free radical hits to every cell of their bodies every day. That's like being shot all day by a free radical machine gun. My friends, we simply weren't designed to take that kind of abuse!

Once again, I must be as clear as possible in the hopes this information will not be misquoted or misused. I want you to eat fresh raw natural foods as much as you can. I want you to avoid things and places that cause oxidative stress, like cigarette smoke and enclosed environments that concentrate toxins. Proper antioxidant nutrients lower cancer risk and slow the aging process, but... **You are an individual, completely unique from all others in the human race. If you do everything right and take the best antioxidant as determined by your genetic makeup, minimize the toxin exposure in** your life, help raise the air quality standard where you live and actively nourish and support your immune system, you may still develop a cancer. There are no guarantees except one–if you do nothing to protect yourself, it is only a matter of time before toxins and stress take their toll on you. Remember what Ben Franklin said, "An ounce of prevention is worth a pound of cure." Old Ben lived in a much cleaner world with much better food, so let's adjust that for today to a *Metric Ton of Cure*!

Epidemiological studies have shown that diets rich in fruits and vegetables, which contain substantial amounts of antioxidant nutrients, protect from the development of many diseases and prolong life.[58] Green leafy vegetables help to protect the body against lung and stomach cancer. Broccoli, brussels sprouts and cauliflower help to protect the body from bowel and thyroid cancer. Garlic, onion, citrus and tomatoes help to protect the body against lung, stomach and bladder cancer.[61] The problem is who can eat enough volume of these foods to get the protection they need?

I have previously mentioned the pilot survey conducted by an oncologist named Dr. Glen Hyland, reported in 1999. The only supplements participants took were the glyconutrient complex detailed in chapter 9 and a phytonutrient complex made from twelve different vegetables and fruits. That complex included phytochemicals from broccoli, brussels sprouts, cabbage, carrot, cauliflower, garlic, kale, onion, tomato, turnip, papaya and pineapple.[62]

Many oncologists fear that anything with antioxidant properties will be contraindicated in chemo- or radiation therapies. Safety must of course always be the first consideration, but once oncologists have been educated in this area not only will they probably no longer fear them, they may join the ranks of doctors who are now recommending them. In addition to Dr. Hyland's work there are at least two other papers of interest regarding safety, one by a Hall and Boyd on improved tolerance to standard cancer therapies while using glyconutrients.[63] The second is by Gardiner, which is specifically on the pharmacokinetics and safety of glyconutritionals.[64]

It makes perfect sense that oncologists would fear using antioxidants especially if they rely on those beta-carotene studies I listed above. Those studies ever scare those who are pro vitamins. But, as mentioned earlier, beta-carotene is not the best way to judge antioxidants overall. Dr. Hyland found that the standard treatment was not neutralized by dietary supplements containing antioxidants and micronutrients. In addition, he found that taking glyconutrients and phytonutrients actually helped the effects of the radiation and the chemotherapy treatments. Another major advantage for these cancer patients was that normal healthy cells, bone marrow, liver and kidneys, as well as mucosal basal cells, were protected from the damage that can be caused by radiation and chemotherapy.

An additional benefit is that malignancies previously non-responsive to therapy (such as sarcomas) responded to this combination of glyconutrients, phytonutrients and chemo- and/or radiation therapy. Also extremely important for patients was that their quality of life while having the treatment improved significantly while taking glyconutrients and phytonutrients during their standard cancer treatments. His was a pilot survey, but it was very encouraging and should open the door for clinical studies.

Supplementing Antioxidants a "Must"

If you still believe that you can just change your diet and eat enough food to get the antioxidant strength you need every day to protect you, you are sadly mistaken. As discussed in an earlier chapter but definitely worth repeating, Dr. Les Packer of the University of California at Berkeley gives us another example of the problem. He studied vitamin E, a well-known and validated antioxidant. He says it would take 100 pounds of liver per day, or 125 tablespoons of peanut butter oil per day, to get the daily amount of vitamin E you need.[62] That's only one antioxidant and the most recent studies show that you need a synergistic complex of antioxidants and their cofactors in complex for optimal antioxidant protection so just how much food do you think you can eat? There is a reason we become less health as a species each year, things have changed. The pristine world we were designed to live on no longer exists.

Doctors or government officials who tell you that if you eat right you can protect yourself from disease are simply behind the times. They do not understand or realize the gravity of the situation that exists today.

I must confess at this point that I have only just revealed the tip of the proverbial iceberg in this book. And if I may carry the metaphor one step further, we are all passengers on the same ship and must work together NOW if we are to stay afloat!

Oxidative stress is not only the principal cause of many diseases such as cancers and heart disease. It also the principal cause of premature aging and all of those unpleasant system breakdowns associated with aging. Since the largest segment of the population is now over 50 and most of them want to hang onto their youth as long as possible the interest in anti aging technologies is perhaps at its highest level ever. Researchers have looked around the world and found that antioxidants can help slow the aging process.[65] The maximum life span for humans that can be documented is 122 years of age. (Personally, I am aiming for 123.)

Living Longer, But Not Necessarily Better

Occasionally I will deliver a presentation on this subject, and someone in the audience who desperately wants to believe that this information is incorrect, or that he or she might be an exception, will say at this point, "Well, if everything is so bad, than why do we live longer now?" That question would be valid only if you did not understand the full scope of this text. But since there will inevitably be a few who don't understand, I will address the question.

In past millennia the principal causes of premature death were violence, accidents, poor sanitation and starvation (usually in that order). During the time of the Roman Empire, for example, the average age was 28. Yet there were those who lived into their 70s and even longer. It was a brutal age that spanned nearly 1,000 years. The Romans had the best sanitation in history until that Empire fell, and the Dark Ages began a time when all previous knowledge and achievements were lost. It was not until the mid-20th century that we regained that full knowledge, and even now in the 21st century there are still nations with less efficient sanitation than that of ancient Rome.

The Romans had constant supplies of clean, fresh water (even hot and cold running water in the more affluent homes), a truly magnificent sewage system (which our own is modeled after), flushing toilets and ample availability of public bath houses that all citizens could use free of charge. Modern health spas are modeled after the Roman baths, which had exercise areas with weights, locker rooms and social gathering areas. Sanitation was not an issue. So outbreaks of disease, although they did happen occasionally, were relatively rare in the Roman world and even less than for some countries today. In addition, food was typically well supplied, but violence was a way of life.

In the 21st century, countries that have solved the problems of sanitation, wholesale violence and starvation have significantly increased life spans, but still living over 100 is rare and even more rare to be healthy at the age. Average life spans were 35 or 40 years of age at the end of the 18th century. By 1900, average life expectancy had increased in the United States to an average of 43. According to a document published by the U.S. Public Health Service in 1953, the average life span had moved up to a whopping 51 years of age average for both males and females. By 1990, the average age had moved into the low- to mid-70's for males and females respectively. As of the year 2000, the latest statistics show the average life span in the U.S. to be about 76.9 years–more specifically, 74.1 for males and 79.5 for females. Still not over 100, however. How many people over 40 in the modern world are there who are not taking at least one pharmaceutical drug daily? How many people over 40 have been saved from death by medical intervention after contracting a disease, infection or having an accident? No, my friends, the facts that the environment is not better and people living longer life spans is not what it seems on the surface.

As medical intervention continues to improve, these statistics will undoubtedly increase marginally. If we consider longevity in just a few modern nations, we can see as an example that Japan and Australia now average approximately 80 and Canada is close to that figure. But the United States–which is all too often the first to recommend synthetics and the last to realize the importance of nature's balance–comes in fourth.[66]

A cautionary note here: Don't be quick to attribute these results to any one single factor. In each country there are many factors in play. In Japan, as they slowly and unfortunately adopted more U.S. foods and habits, their disease rates have gone up. The Australian and Canadian numbers also have many people included who are either recent immigrants who have followed and continue to follow more natural, traditional diets. These are mostly first generation Asians. Subtract their numbers and the longevity stats drop.

The 1990 U.S. census showed that "baby boomers" have been taking over. The number of Americans over 65 years old has more than doubled since 1950 and, from 1980 to 1990, jumped from 25.5 million to 31.1 million. Medical science has played a huge role in keeping people alive–people who under normal conditions would have died much younger.

But being alive and enjoying the optimal quality of life are not necessarily the same. Pharmaceutical drugs and all manner of medical interventions are indeed extending our life spans. But wouldn't it be more desirable to live a better quality of life so that your golden years will be truly golden, not just gold-plated?

The cultures studied that have the longest lifespans can attribute that to several factors but common to all those groups is the consumption of natural antioxidants. When I talk about living to our potential of 100-122 years of age (or longer according to some) I am not talking about people couldn't sustain their lives without drugs or those in wheel chairs or on oxygen support but rather healthy individuals active individuals whose minds still function normally. These individuals start consuming antioxidants in their food from the moment they are weaned from their mother's breasts. Indeed because their mothers take in antioxidants every day, the babies begin getting antioxidants even before they're born. This explains why people in these cultures live the longest and healthiest lives.

At least two of the long-lived cultures studied including the longest lived on Okinawa consume significant levels of Green tea. Green tea, if not over-processed, provides tremendous antioxidant value as well, and in some regions it is a major contributor to antioxidant health as well as longevity. However, not all of the tea leaf contributes to protection against oxidative stress, in fact some Green tea products sold commercially are void of antioxidant value. The amount of tea you would need to drink to get sufficient protection in today's environment would be ridiculous, if tea were relied upon as the sole source of antioxidants. Also, like any other antioxidant, once exposed to oxygen or heat tea's antioxidant protective qualities begin to decline.

Therefore, I strongly caution against dependence on any one antioxidant source as salvation. Green tea alone can't get the job done. Logically, one must extract only the active antioxidant from the green tea, leaving all else behind, and then combine it synergistically with other powerful antioxidants into a complex.

Citrus plays an extremely important role in the diets of the longest-lived people, as do wine and grapes. Fresh citrus (not canned or cooked) should be consumed daily by all, but it simply isn't enough these days by itself.

The skin of the grapes–not the meat or the seeds–provides the most antioxidant value. That is why most antioxidant experts recommend red wine rather than white or blush. Red wines are made from grapes with the skin included. That's where huge amounts of antioxidants are available. If your excuse for drinking white wines is that reds contain sulfites, then I am about to rob you of your excuse. In nature there is something to balance nearly everything that is also natural. If you have sufficient amounts of a trace mineral called molybdenum in your body when you consume red wine, than it will negate the sulfites to a significant extent. It appears that <u>sulfite sensitivity</u> may be caused by a relative deficiency of the <u>enzyme</u> *sulfite oxidase* which breaks down sulfites and requires <u>molybdenum</u> as a <u>co-factor</u>. So symptoms such as nearly instant headaches will be far less frequent if at all. Molybdenum is the principal reason that some enjoy a glass of red and others curse it. Let's be clear: I am not saying load up on molybdenum and then drink a bottle of red wine. Use common sense. The average adult male can tolerate up to four glasses of wine daily, and the average female two. On average, males have a better physical tolerance for alcohol, but that does not mean they should push the envelope. One glass of red wine daily can be therapeutic for adults, unless of course they have certain health conditions that would preclude consuming red wine. Drinking more than one glass a day needs to be considered on an individual basis with all factors taken into account. Always use common sense!

(By the way, I am not advocating drinking red wine. Consuming alcohol is an issue of personal choice. I enjoy a glass of red wine occasionally, but never to excess nor on any regular basis.)

Don't Forget Your Vitamin C

Vitamin C is necessary for more than 300 functions in the human body, and not just as an antioxidant. It is interesting to note that only primates and guinea pigs are unable to manufacture vitamin C on their own, which is why it is an essential vitamin for us.

Vitamin C is known scientifically as ascorbic acid. The makers of synthetic ascorbic acid will cite data that says their product is as effective as natural vitamin C. Medical schools also teach that synthetic ascorbic acid yields the same result as whole, natural vitamin C. However, we have a communications problem here–we need to compare oranges to oranges, if you will.

If you were to extract only ascorbic acid from an orange and compare it to synthetic ascorbic acid, it will be virtually the same. But nature doesn't isolate vitamins like that. For example, just as it is more effective to give the whole vitamin E molecule with all tocopherols and tocotrienol (that piggy-back on vitamin E in nature) rather than just d-alpha tocopherol (normally called vitamin E), it is also more effective to give the whole vitamin C molecule with all of its molecular co-factors.

The factors that occur naturally with ascorbic acid are various flavonoids. Before you go to your favorite nutrition guru's Web site and start splitting hairs about flavonoids, bioflavonoids, flavones, etc., let me save you the trip.

The word flavonoid describes a broad class of water-soluble plant phytochemicals. Flavonoids are more often defined as plant pigments. In fact, the root of the word is from the Latin word *flavus*, which means yellow. Flavones are yellow. (Please recall our earlier discussion about riboflavin {B2} turning your urine yellow.)

Flavonoids are generally broken down into categories, though the experts do not agree universally on how to divide them. One system breaks flavonoids into isoflavones, anthocyanidins, flavans, flavonols, flavones and flavanones.[67] Some of the best-known flavonoids–such as genistein in soy and quercetin in onions–can be considered subcategories of these categories. Although they are all structurally related, their functions are different. Flavonoids also include hesperidin, rutin, citrus flavonoids, plus a variety of others.

Originally flavonoids were labeled as vitamin P. Later, however, it was shown that flavonoids were not separate vitamins but rather co-factors to vitamin C. One of the most recent studies (at the time of this printing) indicates that high single ingredient doses are not as effective as nutrients with their synergist co-factors. Ascorbic acid alone, while definitely helpful, is unlikely to be the best choice. Many papers support the idea that flavonoids and vitamin C combined are more effective and may be required in lower amounts than either nutrient would be in isolation.[68-73]

The key is natural vitamin C complex, not isolated synthetic ascorbic acid. Studies comparing natural versus synthetic sources of beta-carotene and vitamin C have shown that the natural sources are absorbed better, are more bioavailable, and have greater functional activity than the synthetic versions.[73-75]

The Nutrition Desk Reference states, "Natural vitamin C that contains bioflavonoids may have advantages over the synthetic form of vitamin C... Bioflavonoids have been shown to improve the utilization and storage of vitamin C."[76]

Most vitamin C products are made with synthetic ascorbic acid since it is very cheap to mass-produce. The outdated but unfortunately prevailing point of view is that synthetic is no different from natural C. Ironically, drug companies manufacture nearly all ascorbic acid. I would rather have five milligrams of the whole vitamin C molecule with all its natural co-factors than 500 milligrams of ascorbic acid. When I was in practice, natural C with its co-factors was nearly always more effective than ascorbic acid alone. *With antioxidants, more isn't necessarily better since synergy is the key.*

In the last chapter, we discussed glyconutrients as essential for cell-to-cell communication and immune modulation. To defend your cells, glyconutrients, vitamins and minerals are all necessary. To restore, repair and to actually heal your body, glyconutrients, vitamins and minerals are also necessary. But to protect your cells from the effects of our environment and other stresses, you must have antioxidants.

More than three years of continuing research into individual antioxidants resulted in some astonishing data. These antioxidants included flavonoids and vitamins, as well as mineral synergists and substances from various fruits and vegetables. All of these were checked individually and in combination–checked for synergy, checked for levels and checked for the number of milligrams as well as ratios, one to another.[77]

This study initially ran tests using traditional methods that I will discuss in a moment. Then the best combinations as proven by these lab tests were subsequently tested with human subjects.

The Most Accurate Antioxidant Test

There are many methods for testing antioxidant potential, but the most common method in the dietary supplement industry is called ORAC$_{fl}$. ORAC stands for oxygen radical absorption capacity. FL stands for fluorescence. You have to start somewhere in your research, and there needs to be a clear standard so that you can repeat conditions of your experiment. Otherwise it's not really science. So the various ORAC tests offer a set of standards. However, there are a number of flaws to the industry standard for testing antioxidant value. One is that it gives ratings based on fluorescence, and some antioxidants simply don't fluoresce.

Another flaw is that ORAC$_{fl}$ is not the best choice for testing fat-soluble antioxidants. It is more efficient in testing water-soluble antioxidants. Vitamin E is fat-soluble. So how do scientists know that vitamin E is an antioxidant? It has been tested in human blood by something called serum ORAC$_{\beta}$PE. To me, serum ORAC$_{\beta}$PE is the "acid test," if you will. My second choice is testing urine for lipid hydroperoxide, alkenals and 8-OHdG levels, all of which are markers of oxidative damage to lipids and DNA.

As of the time of this printing _any test_ other than serum ORAC$_{\beta}$PE just cannot give you a complete and accurate indicator of your total antioxidant protection. The urine test mentioned above is a helpful adjunct. Still, only serum analysis is fully current and complete. Since the serum ORAC test isn't readily available, other methods are used.

Scientists and entrepreneurs are looking for new ways to test for antioxidant protection because they know that antioxidants are the most important factors for human health in the 21st century. Any form of testing that can point you in the right general direction is a positive thing, as long as it is not misused or misrepresented. Testing a single antioxidant or antioxidant precursor like beta-carotene or co-factors like flavonoids in isolation are incomplete methods for assessing the true protection level in your blood, and therefore may be misleading. You need protection within your body, and any testing outside of the body (although a possible indicator) is simply insufficient. If you test one factor, you learn only about that one factor. Anything else must be inferred and is not definitive.

To ensure that I am not misunderstood on this issue, I'll say it a different way: I am not opposed to testing methods that are less current, less complete or less efficient than serum ORAC$_{\beta}$PE. I simply caution the patient and the healthcare practitioner not to falsely believe that any test less than serum ORAC$_{\beta}$PE will provide an accurate or definitive conclusion about your body's level of protection from oxidative stress. Any test used by any practitioner needs to be clearly understood as to its limitations, and therefore the implications of its findings.

The list of ingredients you see below represents those that were tested individually and found to have the best individual reactions (as of the time of this printing).
1. Complete natural vitamin E
2. Green tea
3. Quercetin (flavonoids)
4. Grape skin extract
5. Complete natural vitamin C

They also show the best synergistic quality when mixed in the appropriate ratio. It is the synergy of these ingredients, not the level of milligrams, that counts. Megadosing when it comes to antioxidants represents simply bad, outdated science.

You may recall that the original recommendation for antioxidant support from food was for each American to eat between two to four servings of fruit, and three to five servings of vegetables, every day. In 2001, the National Academy of Sciences said that Americans were getting 50% less of certain antioxidant nutrients from food than had previously been thought. They therefore recommended doubling the daily intake of fruits and vegetables.[78]

With the data presented in this book, can you believe that even 5-10 servings of fresh raw fruits and vegetables would give you enough antioxidant protection? Sorry, but here I must remain firm: Even grazing on fruits and veggies all day simply can't give you what you need to cope with today's environmental challenges.

The U.S. Department of Agriculture tested fruits and vegetables for serum ORAC value. They had test subjects consume fruits and vegetables from the usual five (up to an experimental ten) servings a day. They found that this increase did significantly boost serum ORAC protection up to 13% after only two weeks.[79] However, in the study using the new synergistic glyconutritional antioxidant blend, using only one 500mg capsule daily raised the serum ORAC$_\beta$PE protection to 19.1%.[20] *That one little capsule offered approximately 47% more protection than eating ten servings of fruits and vegetables.* The test, conducted on healthy subjects, found the peak antioxidant effect for them was at two 500mg capsules daily. That resulted in serum ORAC$_\beta$PE of 37.4%, which is about 300% better than five additional servings of raw fruits and vegetables.

In today's toxic world, dietary supplements are no longer a luxury. Yes, we are living longer, but we are also dying longer. Medical intervention is extending our lives, but only so that we may suffer the ravages of oxidative stress longer. As we age in today's society, we simply increase our probability of suffering from degenerative disease. Heart disease, cancer, stroke, diabetes, Alzheimer's dementia, Parkinson's disease, arthritis, macular degeneration and more than twenty other disease conditions related to oxidative stress are what most of us can look forward to if we are kept alive (though not truly healthy) by improved sanitation, medical intervention and avoidance of death by violence or accidents.

My friends, it is time to face reality if you wish to achieve and maintain true wellness. For real optimal health, you must take the steps outlined in this book for your personal environment and you must take the right dietary supplements every day.

The next chapter will discuss what you can do to make your home and office safer places, as well as some simple actions you can take to help our world survive. If we all work together, not only can we survive–we can even thrive!

References
1. Davies KJ. Oxidative stress: the paradox of aerobic life. *Biochem Soc Symp.* 1995; 61:1-31.
2. Christen Y. Oxidative stress and Alzheimer's disease. *Am J Clin Nutr* 2000;71:621S-629S.
3. Bankson DD, Kestin M, Rifai N. Role of free radicals in cancer and atherosclerosis. *Clin Lab Med.* 1993;13(2):463-480.
4. Harding KL, Judah RD, Gant C. Outcome-based comparison of Ritalin versus food-supplement-treated children with ADHD. *Altern Med Rev.* 2003 Aug;8(3):319-330.
5. Learning Disability Association of America. Top Child Health Agencies Urge Testing to Protect Early Brain Development From Toxins: One Out of Six Affected. New York, Jan. 22 /PRNewswire.
6. Rice DC. Parallels between attention deficit hyperactivity disorder and behavioral deficits produced by neurotoxic exposure in monkeys. *Environ Health Perspect.* 2000;108 (Suppl 3):405-408.
7. Kidd PM. Attention deficit/hyperactivity disorder (ADHD) in children: rationale for its integrative management. *Altern Med Rev.* 2000;5(5):402-28.
8. Lawler JM, Powers SK. Oxidative stress, antioxidant status, and the contracting diaphragm. *Can J Appl Physiol.* 1998;23(1):23-55.
9. Wong A, Dukic-Stefanovic S, Gasic-Milenkovic J, et al. Anti-inflammatory antioxidants attenuate the expression of inducible nitric oxide synthase mediated by advanced glycation end-products in murine microglia. *Eur J Neurosci.* 2001;14(12): 1961-1967.
10. Teixeira S. Bioflavonoids: proanthocyanidins and quercetin and their potential roles in treating musculoskeletal conditions. *J Orthop Sports Phys Ther.* 2002;32(7):357-363.
11. Asha Devi S, Prathima S, Subramanyam MV. Dietary vitamin E and physical exercise: I. Altered endurance capacity and plasma lipid profile in aging rats. *Exp Gerontol.* 2003;38(3):285-290.
12. Reid MB, Stokic DS, Koch SM, et al. N-acetylcysteine inhibits muscle fatigue in humans. *J Clin Invest.* 1994;94(6):2468-2474.
13. Watson JP, Jones DE, James OF, et al. Case report: oral antioxidant therapy for the treatment of primary biliary cirrhosis: a pilot study. *J Gastroenterol Hepatol.* 1999; 14(10):1034-1040.
14. Ball LJ, Birge SJ. Prevention of brain aging and dementia. *Clin Ger Med.* 2002; 18(3):485-503.
15. McDaniel MA, Maier SF, Einstein GO. Brain-specific nutrients: a memory cure? *Nutrition.* 2003;19(11-12):957-975.
16. Galli RL, Shukitt-Hale B, Youdim KA, Joseph JA. Fruit polyphenolics and brain aging: nutritional interventions targeting age-related neuronal and behavioral deficits. *Ann NY Acad Sci.* 2002;959:128-132.
17. Morris MC, Evans DA, Bienias JL, et al. Vitamin E and cognitive decline in older persons. *Arch Neurol.* 2002;59(7):1125-1132.
18. Saliou C, Kitazawa M, McLaughlin L, et al. Antioxidants modulate acute solar ultraviolet radiation-induced NF-kappa-B activation in a human keratinocyte cell line. *Free Radl Biol Med.* 1999;26(1-2):174-183.
19. Koepke CM, Le L, McAnalley S, et al. Results of clinical trials with antioxidants: a review. *GlycoScience & Nutrition.* 2003;4(3):1-7.
20. Boyd S; Gary K; Koepke CM; et al. An open-label pilot study of the antioxidant effect in healthy people of Ambrotose AO™. *GlycoScience & Nutrition* 2003:4(6)1-6.

21. Arthur JR, Nicol F, Beckett GJ. Selenium deficiency, thyroid hormone metabolism, and thyroid hormone deiodinases. *Am J Clin Nutr.* 1993;57(2 Suppl):236S-239S

22. Arthur JR. The role of selenium in thyroid hormone metabolism. *Can J Physiol Pharmacol.* 1991;69(11):1648-1652.

23. Rayman MP, Rayman MP. The argument for increasing selenium intake. *Proc Nutr Soc.* 2002;61(2):203-215.

24. Columbia Encyclopedia, Sixth Edition, New York: Columbia University Press, 2001-04

25. Merrill AH Jr, Henderson JM, Wang E, et al. Metabolism of vitamin B_6 by human liver. *J Nutr.* 1984;114(9):1664-1674.

26. Seelig MS. Auto-immune complications of D-penicillamine--a possible result of zinc and magnesium depletion and of pyridoxine inactivation. *Am Coll Nutr.* 1982;1(2): 207-14.

27. University of Indiana medical biochemistry database: web.indstate.edu/thcme/ mwking /vitamins.html

28. Das UN. Nutrients, essential fatty acids and prostaglandins interact to augment immune responses and prevent genetic damage and cancer. *Nutrition.* 1989;5(2): 106-10.

29. DeRitter E, Bauernfeind JC;. Foods considered for nutrient addition: juices and beverages. *Nutrient Additions to Foods.* Food and Nutrition Press, Inc.; Trumball, CT, 1991.

30. Sillanpää M. *Micronutrients and the nutrient status of soils: a global study.* Werner Söderström Osakeyhtiö; Finland, 1980.

31. Culp FB, Copenhavr JE. The loss of iron, copper, and manganese from vegetables cooked by different methods. *J Home Economics.* 1935; 27: 308-313.

32. DeRitter E;. Foods considered for nutrient addition: dairy products. *Nutrient Additions to Foods.* Bauernfeind JC; Lachance PA, eds. Food and Nutrition Press, Inc; Trumball CT, 1991.

33. Skrede G . Fruits. *Freezing Effects on Food Quality.* Jeremiah LE, ed. Marcel Dekker, Inc.; New York, NY, 1996.

34. Arias R, Lee T, Specca D, Janes H. Quality comparison of hydroponic tomatoes (Lycopersicon esculentum) ripened on and off the vine. *J Food Sci.* 2000; 65: 545-548.

35. Christian J. Charts: Nutrient changes in vegetables and fruits, 1951 to 1999. CTV ca. http://www.ctv.ca/servlet/ArticleNews/story/CTVNews/20020705/favaro_nutrients_chart_020705/Health/story

36. Mayer A-M. Historical changes in the mineral content of fruits and vegetables. *Brit Food J.* 1997;96(6):207-211.

37. Ramberg J, McAnalley BH. From the farm to the kitchen table: a review of the nutrient losses in foods. *GlycoScience & Nutrition.* 2002;3(5):1-12.

38. Howard LA, Wong AD, Perry AK, et al. B-carotene and ascorbic acid retention in fresh and processed vegetables. *J Food Sci.* 1999;64(5):929-936.

39. Kopas-Lane LM, Warthesen JJ. Carotenoid photostability in raw spinach and carrots during cold storage. *J Food Sci.* 1995;60(4):773-776.

40. Demling RH, DeBiasse MA. Micronutrients in critical illness. *Crit Care Clin.* 1995;11(3):651-673.

41. Micronutrient Initiative and UNICEF. Vitamin and Mineral Deficiency: A Global Progress Report, 24 March 2004.

42. Arthur JR. Selenium supplementation: does soil supplementation help and why? *Proc Nutr Soc.* 2003;62(2):393-397.

43. Kang JO. Chronic iron overload and toxicity: clinical chemistry perspective. *Clin Lab

Sci. 14(3):209-219.

44. Fraga CG, Oteiza PI. Iron toxicity and antioxidant nutrients. *Toxicol.* 2002;180(1): 23-32.

45. Dean BS. Krenzelok EP. Multiple vitamins and vitamins with iron: accidental poisoning in children. *Vet Human Toxicol.* 1988;30(1):23-25, 1988.

46. Morris CC. Pediatric iron poisonings in the United States. *South Med J.* 2000;93(4): 352-358.

47. Rimm EB, Stampfer MJ, Ascherio A, et al. Vitamin E consumption and the risk of coronary heart disease in men. *N Engl J Med.* 1993; 328: 1450-1456.

48. Stampfer MJ, Hennekens CH, Manson JE, et al. Vitamin E consumption and the risk of coronary disease in women. *N Engl J Med.* 1993; 328: 1444-1449.

49. Panel on Dietary Antioxidants and Related Compounds. Dietary Reference Intakes for Vitamin C, Vitamin E, Selenium, and Carotenoids Food and Nutrition Board: 2000.

50. The Alpha-Tocopherol, Beta Carotene Cancer Prevention Study Group. The effect of vitamin E and beta carotene on the incidence of lung cancer and other cancers in male smokers. *N Engl J Med.* 1994;330:1029-1035.

51. Omenn GS, Goodman GE, Thornquist MD, et al. Effects of a combination of beta carotene and vitamin A on lung cancer and cardiovascular disease. *N Engl J Med.* 1996;334:1150-1155.

52. Hennekens CH, Buring JE, Manson JE, et al. Lack of effect of long-term supplementation with beta carotene on the incidence of malignant neoplasms and cardiovascular disease. *N Engl J Med.* 1996;334:1145-1149.

53. Greenberg ER, Baron JA, Tosteson TD, et al. A clinical trial of antioxidant vitamins to prevent colorectal adenoma. *N Engl J Med.* 1994;331:141-147.

54. Zhang P, Omaye ST. Beta-carotene and protein oxidation: effects of ascorbic acid and alpha-tocopherol. *Toxicology.* 2000;146:37-47.

55. Zhang P, Omaye ST. Antioxidant and pro-oxidant roles for beta-carotene, alpha-tocopherol and ascorbic acid in human lung cells. *Toxicol In Vitro.* 2001;15:13-24.

56. Palozza P, Calviello G, Serini S, et al. Beta-carotene at high concentrations induces apoptosis by enhancing oxy-radical production in human adenocarcinoma cells. *Free Radic Biol Med.* 2001; 30: 1000-1007.

57. Palozza P, Luberto C, Calviello G, et al. Antioxidant and pro-oxidant role of beta-carotene in murine normal and tumor thymocytes. *Free Radic Biol Med.* 1997;22: 1065-1073.

58. McAnalley BH, Vennum E, Ramberg J, et al. Antioxidants: consolidated review of potential benefits. *GlycoScience & Nutrition.* 2004;5(1):1-21.

59. Barhoumi R, Burghardt RG, Busbee DL, et al. Enhancement of glutathione levels and protection from chemically inititated glutathione depletion in rat liver cells by glyconutritionals. *Proc Fisher Inst Med Res.* 1997;1(1):12-16.

60. Packer L, Colman C. *The Antioxidant Miracle.* John Wiley & Sons, Inc. New York, 1999.

61. Lambert N. Health and food choice. Institute of Food Research, 1999. http://www. ifr.ac.uk/safety/consumerperception.html

62. Hyland G, Miller D. A pilot survey: standard cancer therapy combined with nutraceutical dietary supplementation improves treatment responses and patient quality of life. *Oral Presentation: Comprehensive Cancer Care II: Integrating Complementary & Alternative Therapies in Crystal City, Arlington, VA.*

63. Hall J, Boyd S. Case report: improved tolerance of cancer therapy in a patient taking glyconutritional supplementation. *GlycoScience & Nutrition.* 2002;3(2):1-4.

64. Gardiner T. Pharmacokinetics and safety of glyconutritional sugars for use as dietary supplements. 2004;5(2):1-6.
65. Leaf A;. Every day is a gift when you are over 100. *National Geographic, 2002.*
66. *Encarta Encyclopedia*: http://encarta.msn.com/
67. Peterson J, Dwyer J. Taxonomic classification helps identify flavonoid-containing foods on a semiquantitative food frequency questionnaire. *J Am Diet Assoc* 1998; 98:682–685.
68. Bentsath A, Rusenyak St, Szent-Gyorgyi A. Vitamin nature of flavones. *Nature.* 1936;798.
69. Rusznyak St., Szent-Gyorgyi A. Vitamin P: Flavanols as vitamins. *Nature.* 1936; 133:27.
70. Ambrose AM, De Eds F. The value of rutin and quercetin in scurvy. *J Nutr.* 1949; 38:305-317.
71. Kandaswami C, Perkins E, Soloniuk DS, et al. Ascorbic acid-enhanced antiprolifera-tive effect of flavonoids on squamous cell carcinoma *in vitro. Anticancer Drugs.* 1993;4(1):91-96.
72. Vrijsen R, Everaert L, Boeye A. Antiviral activity of flavones and potentiation by ascorbate. *J Gen Virol.* 1988;69(Pt 7):1749-1751.
73. Vinson JA, Bose P. Comparative bioavailability to humans of ascorbic acid alone or in a citrus extract. *Am J Clin Nutr.* 1988;48(3):601-604.
74. Ben-Amotz A, Levy Y. Bioavailability of a natural isomer mixture compared with syn-thetic all-trans beta-carotene in human serum. *Am J Clin Nutr.* 1996;63(5):729-734.
75. Vinson, J. A. and P. Bose. Comparative bioavailability of synthetic and natural vita-min C in guinea pigs. *Nutr Rep Int.* 27:875-880.
76. Garrison RH, Somer E. *The Nutrition Desk Reference.* Keats Publishing, Inc.; New Canaan, CT, 1990.
77. McAnalley B, Gardiner T, Summey A, et al. Innovations in the development of a superior antioxidant: Ambrotose AO™. *Mannatech R&D Report.* 2004;1(1):1-7.
78. Panel of Micronutrients. Dietary reference intakes for vitamin A, vitamin K, arsenic, boron, chromium, copper, iodine, iron, manganese, molybdenum, nickel, silicon, vanadium, and zinc. Food and Nutrition Board: 2001.
79. Cao G, Booth SL, Sadowski JA, et al. Increases in human plasma antioxidant capacity after consumption of controlled diets high in fruit and vegetables. *Am J Clin Nutr.* 1998;68(5):1081-1087.

Chapter 11
Dealing with Household Toxins

Up to this point, I have been discussing problems with our environment and the threats they pose to our health. The previous two chapters explained what you can do in terms of nutritional self-help. The following chapters offer brief facts and quick tips about how to make your home and our world a safer place.

This chapter and the two that follow cover toxins in your home and how you can reduce their threat to you and your family. There will be some interesting, natural tips you can use for your safety and to improve the health of our planet as well. We will look at common chemicals, including pesticides in the home and how you can protect against their harmful effects. I will also provide "recipes" for natural, non-toxic cleaners and pesticides you can make yourself. Then I will discuss some shocking information about the air quality in your home, but I will also give you some practical tips on how to effectively cope.

Finally, I will discuss both water quality and water conservation issues. You'll be surprised to learn just how little clean water there is and how much is wasted every day.

You will be amazed to find out how much impact <u>you</u> can personally make on the health of our world. You are more important than you may realize. Your efforts as a single individual can and will make a huge difference in the fate of our planet.

Your Home–More Toxic Than You May Realize[1]
- The average American home contains 3-10 gallons of hazardous materials.
- The average household typically uses and stores more than 60 hazardous products, including household cleaners, automotive products, paints, solvents and pesticides.
- In 1999, 2.1 million human poisonings were reported to poison control centers in the United States. More than 50 percent of these cases involved children under the age of five.
- The U.S. government has not conducted even basic toxicity testing for about 75 percent of the 15,000 high-volume chemicals in commercial use. Also, more than 90 percent of these high-volume chemicals have not been tested for specific health effects on children.
- EPA studies of human exposure to air pollutants indicate that indoor air levels of many pollutants may be 2-5 times (and occasionally, more than 100 times!) higher than outdoor levels. Cleaning products and other household products are among the many culprits.
- Over 150 chemicals found in the average home have been linked to allergies, birth defects, cancer and psychological abnormalities.

Read Labels Carefully
- The Federal Hazardous Substances Labeling Act (FHSLA, sometimes called the Federal Hazardous Substances Act) requires manufacturers to label active ingredients in household products that are considered "proximate" hazards, but not inert ingredients with chronic (long-term) effects.
- Remember: Warning label advisory words–for example, "DANGER" and "CAU-

TION"–apply only to acute or immediate hazards. Labels do NOT indicate the effect chemicals will have on chronic or long-term health. Thus, degenerative diseases or those with a long latency period are not addressed by advisory words. In addition, product labels are not required to inform consumers of the types of hazards associated with the product.

- A study by the New York Poison Control Center found that 85 percent of product warning labels they studied were inadequate. Some labels contain incorrect first aid information, and others warn against dangers that don't exist.
- The Environmental Protection Agency (EPA) says as much as 90% of a pesticide product is made up of so-called inert ingredients. Supposedly, "inert" means inactive. However, the EPA lists seven inert pesticide ingredients known to be toxic to humans and 94 that are potentially toxic. Since these ingredients are supposedly inert, no warning is required. In fact, they don't even have to be listed on the container. Does your favorite politician know this? Why don't you make sure they do know it? If he or she does know it, why do they allow it?
- The Consumer Product Safety Commission is charged with enforcing the FHSLA, which defines "hazardous substance" as "any substance or mixture of substances that is (i) toxic, (ii) corrosive, (iii) an irritant, (iv) a strong sensitizer, (v) flammable or combustible, or (vi) generates pressure through decomposition, heat or other means, if such substances or mixture of substances may cause substantial personal injury or substantial illness during or as a proximate result of any customary or reasonably foreseeable handling or use, including reasonably foreseeable ingestion by children."

Toxic Household Products

(Source unless noted: U.S. Environmental Protection Agency)[2]

Today, the number of toxins found in the average home is astounding. Things that you wouldn't give a second thought to may be making you sick or even worse. Why are there currently 6.3 million American children with asthma? What chemicals in your home can cause fatigue, dizziness or worse?

This book is intended to alert you to toxic dangers, offer some solutions and move you to take action. It is not meant to be the definitive encyclopedic reference of more than 75,000 potential toxins. I can cover only major or common areas in this chapter–ones that present the gravest threats and the best possible solutions. Let's start by looking in your closet, a place you may never have imagined as being threatening to your health.

Your Closet Can Affect the World

During the dry-cleaning process for your clothes, liquid chemical solvents are used to remove stains from fabrics. In an earlier chapter, we mentioned that the primary chemicals of concern are perchloroethylene, also known as PCE or "Perc". It is also known by the following names: carbon bichloride, carbon dichloride, ethylene tetrachloride, perchlor, Perclene, perk, 1,1,2,2-tetrachloroethylene, and tetrachloroethene. Perc is a colorless liquid with a sharp, sweet odor that evaporates quickly. Perc replaced kerosene and other petroleum-based solvents, which were generally used in dry cleaning's early days.

The EPA estimates there are approximately 30,000 dry cleaners now using Perc nationwide. Improper storage, handling and disposal of Perc–along with other volatile organic compounds used in dry cleaning, such as trichloroethane and trichloroethylene–have resulted in significant contamination of our soil and groundwater. Perc does not bind well to soil, so it may move rapidly through soil and into groundwater, where it does not dissolve completely.

Perc enters the body through inhalation or ingestion and can remain stored in fat tissue. Short-term exposure to Perc can cause adverse health effects to the nervous system, ranging from dizziness, fatigue, headaches and sweating to loss of coordination and unconsciousness. Contact with Perc in liquid or vapor form can irritate the skin, eyes, nose and throat. Long-term exposure to Perc can cause liver and kidney damage. Perc has been shown to cause cancer in laboratory animals that repeatedly inhaled the chemical.

In a study published by the Centers for Disease Control (CDC), 1,708 dry-cleaning workers exposed to Perc had elevated, standardized mortality ratios for tongue, bladder, esophagus, intestine, lung and cervical cancer, plus pneumonia. They also exhibited a statistically significant increase in diseases of the stomach and duodenum.

What Can You Do?[3,4]
- If possible, avoid buying "dry-clean-only" clothes.
- Learn which dry-clean-only garments can be safely washed with non-toxic methods.
- Take your clothes to a "wet-cleaning" facility, whenever possible. Wet cleaning is a process that uses steam and mild soaps instead of toxic solvents.
- If you have clothes dry-cleaned, remove them from the plastic bag as soon as possible and hang them outside or in a ventilated area for a while before wearing them.

Pesticides–They kill more than just pests.
Earlier I spoke of pesticide concentrations typically being 3-5 times and as much as ten times greater in your home than outdoors. Now let's examine this problem in greater detail.

A survey of national pesticide use found that 37 percent of all U.S. households use pesticides even when no significant insect problems exist. Is it really so surprising then that more than 100,000 cases of pesticide exposures have been reported to U.S.-certified regional poison control centers?

Health Effects from Pesticides
Both the active and inert ingredients in pesticides can be organic compounds. Therefore, both can add to the levels of airborne organics inside homes and can cause the types of health issues I address in this book. Unfortunately, we have insufficient understanding at this time about what levels of pesticide concentrations are required to produce these adverse health effects.

However, let's use some common sense: These chemicals cause illness and disease, sometimes resulting in death. They are everywhere, and we must take the proper steps. The presence of even a little poison is never acceptable.

Exposure to high levels of cyclodiene pesticides has been shown to produce various symptoms, including headaches, dizziness, muscle twitching, weakness, tingling sensations and nausea. In addition, the EPA is concerned that cyclodienes might cause long-term damage to the liver and the central nervous system, as well as increased risk of cancer.

No sale or commercial use is currently permitted for the following cyclodiene or related pesticides: chlordane, aldrin, dieldrin and heptachlor. The only exception is the use of heptachlor by utility companies to control fire ants in underground cable boxes.

The following is a list of pesticides and the purposes for which they are commonly used in our homes:
- Algaecides–Control algae in swimming pools and water tanks.
- Antimicrobials–Kill micro-organisms (such as bacteria and viruses).
- Attractants–Contain a pesticide and food to lure insects or rodents inside.
- Disinfectants and sanitizers–Kill disease-producing micro-organisms in the kitchen and bathroom.
- Fumigants–Produce gas or vapor intended to destroy pests in the house or in the ground.
- Fungicides–Kill fungi, including blights, mildews, molds and rusts. Some are no longer effective.
- Herbicides–Kill weeds.
- Insecticides–Kill insects and other arthropods.
- Miticides–Kill mites that feed on plants and animals.
- Microbial pesticides–Micro-organisms that kill or inhibit pests, including insects or other microorganisms. Many are designed to consume the pests' food supply.
- Molluscicides–Kill snails and slugs.
- Nematicides–Kill nematodes (microscopic, worm-like organisms that feed on plant roots).
- Pheromones–Biochemicals that disrupt the mating behavior of insects.
- Repellents–Repel pests, including insects (such as mosquitoes) and birds.
- Rodenticides–Control mice and other rodents.

Depending on the site and pest to be controlled, one or more of the following steps can be effective:
- Use of biological pesticides, such as *Bacillus thuringiensis*, for the control of gypsy moths.
- Selection of disease-resistant plants.
- Frequent washing of indoor plants and pets.

Termite damage can be reduced or prevented by making certain that wooden building materials do not come into direct contact with the soil and by storing firewood away from the home. By appropriately fertilizing, watering and aerating lawns, the need for chemical pesticide treatments of lawns can be dramatically reduced.

If you decide to use a pest control company, choose very carefully. Ask for an inspection of your home and get a written control program for evaluation before you sign any contract. The control program should list specific names of pests to be controlled and chemicals to be used. It should also reflect any of your safety concerns. Insist on references for a proven record of competence and customer satisfaction.

Dispose of unwanted pesticides safely. If you have unused or partially used pesticide containers, dispose of them according to the directions on the label or on special household hazardous waste collection days. If there are no such collection days in your community, work with others to organize them.

Call the National Pesticide Telecommunications Network (NPTN) at 800-858-PEST.

EPA sponsors the NPTN to answer your questions about pesticides and to provide selected EPA publications about pesticides and how to minimize their dangers to human health.

Make your home safer from the dangers of pesticides.

The first answer for almost every problem is simply to use some common sense. That means to avoid using commercial pesticides. Use the safe, natural alternatives listed in this book.

- If you must use chemical pesticides, ventilate the area well after pesticide use.
- Mix or dilute pesticides outdoors or in a well-ventilated area and only in the amounts that will immediately be used.
- If possible, take plants and pets outside when applying pesticides to them.
- Store pesticides outside of your home. (Garage, tool shed, patio, etc.)

Reduce the accumulation of pesticides in your home.

- Remove porous surfaces wherever they are not required. Most pesticides accumulate in carpets although they can collect in any porous material. As stated in an earlier chapter, carpet is the primary storage area for household toxins of all types. Smooth-surfaced floors such as tile or wood do not collect toxins.

- Where you feel you must have carpet, make it the shortest nap available. I love plush carpet as much as anyone, but scientific study shows that the deeper the pile, the more toxin (of virtually every type) that can and will be stored there.[5]

- Use a proven filtration system in your vacuum cleaners. Change or clean these filters at least weekly. Many vacuum cleaners are not very efficient. They may pick up large particles but blow the health-threatening toxins all over the room, where the toxic dust will simply fall back onto the carpet. Perhaps you are fortunate enough to have a central vacuum that exhausts to a filter in your garage, at least one that will get the toxins away from your carpet. Ordinary vacuum bags simply blow toxins around and make things worse. Vacuum bags and filters are a breeding ground for bacteria. They blow bacteria into the air that everyone then breathes. Shop carefully for a new vacuum cleaner.

- Get new doormats and insist that everyone use them. Clean the mats regularly. Again, I urge you to take a lesson from the Japanese and other Eastern cultures and remove your shoes when you enter the home. Insist everyone else does so too. We bring in most of the toxins that collect in our carpets on the bottoms of our shoes. Simply using mats and removing your shoes can reduce the toxin level in your home by a factor of six![5]

What can I do to reduce the need for pesticides?

- After eating, clean all areas thoroughly. Any crumbs or liquids remaining can attract pests. Dirty dishes should be cleaned and put away as soon as possible. Use damp cloths–not cleansers–around the kitchen area unless you have no other choice. Use only natural, non-toxic, citrus-based products that can help you cut grease during cleaning. More natural cleaners are currently being researched.

- Make sure all potential points of pest entry are blocked with caulking or a sealant of some type. If pests can't gain entry to your house, you won't have to worry about killing them. Ensure that door and window jambs also have tight seals. Insects belong outdoors and like it or not they are crucial to the ecosystem. As long as they are not in your home, there are few reasons to go after them.

• Don't let water pool in the sink. Check to make sure you have no plumbing leaks, even where you would not normally look for them. Many pests are attracted to water, so don't leave containers with liquid out.

• For foods that will not be refrigerated, make sure the food containers are sealed tightly. These containers should be made of glass or plastic—preferably glass. When rodents smell food, they will simply gnaw through a box or bag to get to it.

• Since pesticides accumulate in porous material, have smooth surfaces wherever possible.

• Make your own non-toxic natural pesticides, using the recipes below.

Natural Insecticide Recipes To Safely Replace Toxic Chemicals
House and Garden Natural Insecticide
2 tablespoons liquid dish soap
1 quart water
Spray bottle

Mix soap and water. Add to spray bottle. Spray plants evenly, aiming directly at pests whenever possible. Warning, don't spray directly at stinging insects. Although this mix may drive them off it may not in some cases, so don't take chances. Spray the plants while the stinging insects are not present. Insects that eat plants will typically not return, as they will find that sprayed plant distasteful.

General Natural Insecticide
2 cloves of garlic
1 small onion
1 tablespoon cayenne (red) pepper
2 tablespoons liquid dish soap
1 quart warm water

Finely chop onion and garlic. Mix with water and add cayenne pepper. Let sit for one hour, then add dish soap. Mix well. Strain mixture and pour into a spray bottle. Keep refrigerated. Good for 1-2 weeks.

Household Pest Treatments
Ants
Use boric acid, talcum powder or chalk as a barrier along the line of entry.

Roaches
Set out a dish containing equal parts sugar and baking soda. Roaches are attracted to sugar, and baking soda is deadly to them.

Fleas
Peel from 2 large oranges
Peel from 1 grapefruit
2 cloves garlic
1 tablespoon rosemary

1 pint warm water
Combine ingredients in blender set on "liquefy." Heat mixture over low heat for 15 minutes. Strain mixture and pour into a spray bottle. Spray on pet, and massage thoroughly into your pet's coat, avoiding contact with pet's eyes.

Other Common Household Toxics[6]

- *hypochlorite. (chlorine bleach)* Lung and eye irritant. Household bleach is the most common cleaner accidentally swallowed by children. If mixed with ammonia or acid-based cleaners (including vinegar), releases highly toxic chloramine gas. Short-term exposure to chloramine gas may cause mild asthmatic symptoms or more serious respiratory problems.

- *Petroleum distillates.* (metal polishes) Short-term exposure can cause temporary eye clouding. Longer exposure can damage the nervous system, skin, kidneys and eyes.

- *Ammonia.* (glass cleaner) Lung and skin irritant. If mixed with chlorine, releases toxic chloramine gas. Short term exposure to chloramine gas may cause coughing, choking and lung damage. Asthmatics may be particularly vulnerable to asthma and chloramine fumes.

- *Phenol and cresol.* (disinfectants) Corrosive. Can cause diarrhea, fainting, dizziness and kidney/liver damage.

- *Nitrobenzene.* (furniture and floor polishes) Can cause shallow breathing, vomiting and death. Associated with cancer and birth defects.

- *Formaldehyde.* (preservative in many household products; used as a glue in particleboard and plywood furniture). Probable human carcinogen. See details below.

- *Perchloroethylene.* (Perc) or 1-1-1 trichloroethane solvents (dry cleaning fluid, spot removers and carpet cleaners). Discussed in detail earlier in the chapter.

- *Naphthalene or paradichlorobenzene.* (mothballs, toilet bowl cleaners) Naphthalene fumes can irritate eyes, skin and respiratory tract. Chronic exposure to naphthalene can cause damage to liver, kidneys, skin and central nervous system. Paradichlorobenzene is a probable carcinogen that can also harm the central nervous system, liver and kidneys. High concentration of fumes may irritate eyes, nose, throat and lungs.

- *Hydrochloric acid or sodium acid sulfate.* (toilet bowl cleaners) Can either burn the skin or cause vomiting, diarrhea and stomach burns if swallowed. Can cause blindness if inadvertently splashed in the eyes.

- *Phenol and pentachlorophenol.* (spray starch) Any aerosolized particle, including corn-starch, may irritate the lungs.

- *Phosphates.* Minerals that act as water softeners. Although they are very effective cleaners, phosphates also act as fertilizers. When cleaning products go down the drain, phosphates are discharged into rivers, lakes, estuaries and oceans. In lakes and rivers especially, phosphates cause a rapid growth of algae, resulting in pollution of the water. Many states have banned phosphates from household laundry detergents and some other cleaning products. Automatic dishwasher detergents are usually exempt from phosphate restrictions, and most major brands contain phosphates. Some phosphate-free alternatives are available, and hand-dishwashing liquids do not contain phosphates.

- *Alkylphenols and their derivatives.* Found in some laundry detergents, disinfecting cleaners, all-purpose cleaners, spot removers, hair colors and other hair-care products and spermicides.

- *Alkylphenol ethoxylates.* Endocrine (glandular) disruptors. Produced in the environmental breakdown of alkylphenol ethoxylate surfactants, slow to biodegrade and have been shown to disrupt the endocrine systems of fish, birds and mammals. (Humans are mammals.)

- *Volatile organic compounds.* Widely used as ingredients in household products. All of these products can release pollutants as you use them, and, to some degree, while in storage.

EPA's Total Exposure Assessment Methodology (TEAM) studies found levels of about a dozen common organic pollutants to be 2 to 5 times higher inside homes than outside, regardless of whether the homes were located in rural or highly industrial areas. Additional TEAM studies indicate that since people use products containing organic chemicals, they can expose themselves and others to very high pollutant levels. In addition, elevated concentrations can persist in the air long after the activity has been completed.

Many organic compounds are known to cause cancer in animals. and some are suspected of causing–or are known to cause–cancer in humans.

Some of the hazardous volatile organic compounds (VOCs) that frequently pollute indoor air–such as **toluene, styrene, xylenes** and **trichloroethylene**–may be emitted from aerosol products, dry-cleaned clothing, paints, varnishes, glues, art supplies, cleansers, spot removers, floor waxes and polishes, and air fresheners.

- **Trichloroethylene** is one of the chemicals suspected of causing a cluster of childhood leukemia cases due to drinking water contamination in the town of Woburn, Massachusetts in the early 1980s. The subsequent lawsuit against the polluting company was the subject of the 1995 book and 1998 film, **A Civil Action**.

- High levels of **toluene** can put pregnant woman at risk of having babies with neurological problems, retarded growth and developmental problems. **Xylenes** can also cause birth defects.

- **Styrene** is a suspected endocrine disruptor–a chemical that can interfere, block or mimic hormones in humans or animals.

- VOCs such as **xylene, ketones** and **aldehydes** are found in many aerosol products and air fresheners. Researchers found that babies less than six months old in homes where air fresheners are used on most days had 30 percent more ear infections than those exposed less than once a week.

- **Formaldehyde** is a possible human carcinogen. Levels of formaldehyde in air as low as 0.1 ppm (0.1 part formaldehyde per million parts of air) can cause watery eyes, burning sensations in the eyes, nose and throat, stuffy nose, nausea, coughing, chest tightness, wheezing, skin rashes and allergic reactions. Formaldehyde isn't just found in glues, carpet and building materials. It is also generated in the form of a gas produced while dry ink toners are subjected to heat as the machines run. This effect emanates from such commonplace office systems as copy machines. So, if you feel bad at the office, this may be one of the reasons.

- Babies frequently exposed to aerosols had a 22 percent increase in diarrhea, and pregnant women frequently exposed to these products had 25 percent more headaches and a 19 percent increase in postnatal depression compared to those less frequently exposed. Paints, cleaners and other products with no or very low levels of VOCs and other hazardous ingredients are available.

Bleach and Cancer

Chlorine (sodium hypochlorite) is found in paper products such as toilet paper and paper towels. Bleaching paper products with chlorine bleach causes the formation of dioxin, an extremely toxic and persistent chemical known to cause cancer and disrupt the endocrine system.

Deadly Dioxins Proliferate

Dioxin is everywhere in the environment and presents a broad spectrum of threats to you and your family. I must devote some space to this major toxic chemical category and its threats to human life since it is not going away, and you must be aware of how to deal with its presence.

- Dioxin is a highly toxic chemical that accumulates in our environment, our food and bodies. According to the EPA, the average adult already has enough dioxin in their bodies today to cause adverse health effects. It is highly persistent in the environment and extremely resistant to chemical or physical breakdown. The term "dioxin" encompasses a family of 75 chemicals technically known as chlorinated dibenzo dioxins.

Health concerns

- The World Health Organization upgraded dioxin from a "probable" to a "known human carcinogen" in February, 1997, and the U.S. National Institutes of Health followed suit in October 2000.

- Exposure to dioxin has been linked to diabetes, attention deficit disorder, learning disabilities, weakened immune systems, infertility and endometriosis.

- On May 23, 2002 the EPA reported in its "Toxics Release Inventory" (TRI) that 99,814 grams of dioxin were released into the environment in the year 2000. **One gram of dioxin is enough to exceed the acceptable daily intake for more than 40 million people for one year, according to the Stop Dioxin Exposure Campaign.**

Sources and exposure

Dioxins are never manufactured deliberately (except during laboratory research) and are unintentionally created in two principal ways:

- **Heating plastic releases dioxin.** You should never cook in plastic containers. Dioxins are released when materials such as household garbage or toxic waste–including hospital waste, leaded gasoline, plastic, paper and dioxin-contaminated wood–are burned. **Do not microwave plastic containers unless you want your body to work overtime fighting cancer cells.** Remove food from plastic first and put it into glass cookware that is designed for oven, microwave or stove tops. Yes, that includes cling wrap and other "microwaveable plastic wraps. Microwaveable simply means it will not be destroyed by the microwaves and will not cause a reaction with the waves that could harm the oven. It does not take into account the dioxin release from heating plastic. It is likely that no plastics manufacturer or vendor ever knew this danger. If they read this book, they will.

- **Manufacturing processes create dioxins.** These processes are used to make specific pesticides, preservatives, disinfectants and paper products.

The latest TRI data reflects only a fraction of the dioxin that is being released into the environment every day, according to the "Stop Dioxin Exposure Campaign." TRI data does not include a number of dioxin sources, including the largest waste concentrations incinerated by cities, hospitals and rural communities. So, there is no way at present to know the full extent of this threat.

Dioxin pollution is persistent and bioaccumulative, which essentially means that it eventually ends up in our food and bodies. According to "The American People's Dioxin Report," about 90 to 98 percent of the general population's exposure to dioxins is through contaminated food—primarily from eating the animal fat in meat, fish, poultry and dairy products.

Chlorine alternatives
- Chlorine-free toilet paper and paper towels are available at many natural food stores. Additionally, newspaper can be used in place of paper towels for cleaning windows, and rags can be used for other surfaces.

Alternative cleaning products
- Many household cleansers contain chlorine bleach. Chlorine bleach, or sodium hypochlorite, is a lung and eye irritant. If mixed with ammonia or acid-based cleaners (including vinegar), chlorine bleach releases toxic chloramine gas. Short-term exposure to this gas may cause mild asthmatic symptoms or more serious respiratory problems.

To be on the safe side, don't mix chlorine bleach with anything. Just avoid chlorine bleach altogether. The EPA recommends using a non-chlorine bleach, such as hydrogen peroxide, to bleach clothes. (Yes, it will work to get your clothes clean and white! Please give it a try, and see for yourself!)

Eco-friendly Alternatives to Commercial Cleaners and Other Household Products
Eco-friendly alternatives to commercial cleaning products...
- are less polluting to manufacture.
- are less likely, in some cases, to cause injury if accidentally ingested.
- don't cause indoor air pollution in your home.
- are generally less expensive than commercial products.
- can reduce packaging waste.
- are simple and effective and have been used for generations.
- can help you save space in your cupboards and closets.
- are less likely to harm the environment during and after use.

Shopping list:
- Vinegar
- Baking soda
- Corn-starch salt
- Borax **(toxic if ingested)**
- Lemon juice
- Olive oil
- Mild liquid soap (not detergent)
- Reusable steel wool—not commercial cleaning pads that contain toxic cleaners and no sodium hypochlorite

• Use non-chlorine scouring powder

Recipes and Tips:

All-purpose Cleaner

Mix 2 Tbsp baking soda with 1 pint warm water in a spray bottle. Add a squeeze of lemon juice or a splash of vinegar to cut grease.

Surface cleaner

Find a combination that works for you, and always keep some ready in a spray bottle. You'll find that weak acids like vinegar and lemon juice are good at cutting grease. Mix 1 quart hot water, 1 tsp vegetable oil-based soap or vegetable oil-based detergent, 1 tsp borax and 2 Tbsp vinegar.

Note: Vinegar is a mild acid that can be used to cut grease. Borax can be used as a water softener to prevent soapy deposits–especially good in areas with hard water. Alternate options:

• Mix 1/2 cup vinegar in 1 quart of warm water.
• Dissolve baking soda in hot water for a general cleaner.
• For a soft scrubbing paste, mix some baking soda with enough liquid soap to make a paste. Make only as much as you need since it dries quickly.

No-streak glass/window cleaner

• Mix 1/4 cup white vinegar and 1 quart warm water.
• Or mix 1/4 cup white vinegar, 1 Tbsp corn-starch and 1 quart warm water.

Apply with a spray bottle or sponge. Wipe with crumpled newspaper instead of paper towels for lint-free results.

Oven cleaner

Use one of the following methods:

• Mix 1 part vinegar to about 4 parts water. Put into a spray bottle. Spray on cool oven surface. Scrub the oven clean. Use baking soda or a citrus-based cleaner on stubborn spots.
• Mix together in a spray bottle 2 Tbsp liquid soap (not detergent), 2 tsp borax and enough warm water to fill the bottle. Make sure everything is completely dissolved to avoid clogging the squirting mechanism. Spray on mixture, holding the bottle very close to the oven surface. Leave the solution on for 20 minutes, then scrub with steel wool and a non-chlorine scouring powder.
• Use a non-chlorinated scouring powder.
• Use a baking soda, salt and water paste.
• Clean glass oven door with a non-chlorinated scouring powder. Use razor blade or spatula for tough spots.

Notes: Avoid aerosol oven cleaners and cleaners containing lye (sodium hydroxide). Avoid chlorinated scouring powders such as Comet and Ajax. Never use abrasive cleaning materials on self-cleaning ovens. For preventative cleaning, use baking soda dissolved in water.

Non-toxic toilet bowl cleaner

• Pour 1 cup borax and 1/2 cup white vinegar and leave in toilet bowl overnight. Flush to wet the sides. Sprinkle more borax around the toilet bowl, and then drizzle with vinegar. Leave for several hours before scrubbing with a toilet brush.
• For stains in toilet bowl, try a paste of lemon juice and borax. Let it sit about 20

minutes, then scrub with bowl brush.

Notes: Avoid solid toilet bowl deodorizers that contain paradichlorobenzene, which you can easily recognize since it turns your toilet water very blue. There is evidence that this chemical causes cancer in laboratory animals. Some toilet bowl cleaning products contain acids (read labels). If acids are mixed with a cleaner containing chlorine, toxic chloramine gas will be released, so avoid these products.

Tub and sink cleaner
- Use non-chlorinated cleanser.
- For toughest stains, try a citrus-based cleaner at full strength (undiluted).
- Use fine-grain wet/dry sandpaper (400 grit) to remove pot marks in porcelain sinks (gentler than common scouring cleansers).
- To remove mineral deposits around faucets, cover deposits with strips of paper towels soaked in vinegar. Let sit for one hour, then clean.

Note: Hard water means the water has a high mineral content (e.g. calcium, lime, magnesium, iron, etc.). This often results in whitish mineral deposits left on faucets, shower doors, drains and windows. Vinegar, a weak acid, can safely dissolve many of these deposits.

Bleach
- Use hydrogen peroxide-based bleaches. Hydrogen peroxide breaks down to become water and oxygen in wastewater.

Laundry
- For a fabric rinse, add 1/4 cup of vinegar to the washing machine's rinse cycle. This eliminates the scratchy feel of laundered clothes by rinsing detergent completely from clothes.
- Brighten clothes by adding 1/2 cup of lemon juice to the rinse cycle.
- Reduce the amount of laundry detergent per load by adding 1/2 cup of baking soda or borax to the wash.

Dishes
- For hand-washing: Use vegetable oil-based soaps/detergents.
- For automatic dishwasher: Automatic dishwashing detergents typically have a very high level of phosphates. At this time, I know of only one automatic dishwashing detergent that doesn't. Undoubtedly there will be more so read labels carefully before buying.

Unclogging drains
Use one of the following methods:
- Pour one or two handfuls of baking soda down the drain pipe followed by 1/2 cup white vinegar and cover tightly for one minute. The chemical reaction between the two substances will create pressure in the drain and dislodge the obstruction. Rinse with hot water.
- Pour 1/2 cup salt and 1/2 cup baking soda followed by lots of hot water.
- Plunge the sink. For directions, see *Better Homes & Gardens* magazine.
- Use a drain snake–also called a sink auger–to unclog stubborn drains. Drain snakes can be purchased at hardware stores or ordered online, sometimes for less than the cost of a bottle of chemical drain cleaner. More expensive, heavy-duty drain snakes can be rented for less than the cost of many chemical drain cleaners. Learn how to use drain snakes from *Better Homes & Gardens*.
- Read "Unclogging a Sink Drain" on **DoItYourself.com** for various ideas.

Mothballs

- Mothballs are typically blue this because they contain paradichlorobenzene. It is deadly to moths and unlikely to be healthy for us. Cedar (unless you are allergic to it) will cause no harm to you and will not harm any other life either (including moths), but they won't go near it. Store clean clothing in airtight containers or sealed bags with cedar blocks and/or shavings (available as cage bedding in pet stores). Place cedar in drawers and closets as well. Inspect any used clothing or furniture carefully for moths or larvae before bringing them into the house, or clean them first. Vigorously shaking clothes will remove larvae and eggs (remember to vacuum well afterwards). The heat of the dryer will also kill larvae and eggs. (Source: Children's Health Environmental Coalition.)

Floor or furniture polish

- Use one of the following methods: Combine 1 part lemon juice with 2 parts olive oil and apply a thin coat of this liquid. Rub in well with a soft cloth. Mix three parts olive oil and one part vinegar.

Carpet deodorizer

- Sprinkle carpet liberally with baking soda. Wait 15 minutes, then vacuum. For musty rugs that have been sitting in the attic for a while, leave the baking soda overnight.

Metal polishing

- Brass: Mix 1/2 tsp salt and 1/2 cup white vinegar with enough flour to make a paste. Apply thickly. Let sit for 15-30 minutes. Rinse thoroughly with water to avoid corrosion.
- Copper: Polish with a paste of lemon juice and salt.
- Silver: Boil silver 3 minutes in a quart of water containing 1 teaspoon baking soda, 1 teaspoon salt and a piece of aluminum foil. Or rub silver with a baking soda/water paste and a soft cloth. Rinse and polish dry. Or rub silver with toothpaste. Use a toothbrush to clean raised surfaces. Be careful not to scratch surfaces. Be gentle and use a light hand.
- Chrome: Wipe with vinegar, rinse with water and then dry. (Good for removing hard water deposits.) Or shine chrome fixtures with baby oil and a soft cloth. (Good for removing soap scum from faucets.)
- Stainless steel: Clean and polish with a baking soda/water paste or a non-chlorinated scouring powder.

Paper towels and rags

- Crumpled newspaper is a great substitute for paper towels when cleaning windows. If you do use paper towels for cleaning, choose unbleached paper towels with high post-consumer recyclable content. Reusable cloth rags are also a good choice.

Trash Toxics the Right Way

Get rid of toxic household products stored under your kitchen sink and in your basement, but don't pour them down the drain or throw them in the trash. Remember that many household products are considered hazardous waste. Contact your local environmental agency or public works department to find out about hazardous waste disposal in your area. You can read about local disposal rules at **www.cleanup.org**

FOR THIS:	TRY THIS:
Air freshener	Simmer cinnamon and cloves. Leave opened box of baking soda in room or set out a dish of vinegar.
Aluminum spot remover	2 tablespoons cream of tartar and 1 quart hot water.
Car battery corrosion	Baking soda and water.
Cleaners (general household)	Mix 1/2 cup ammonia, 1/3 cup vinegar, 1/4 cup baking soda in one gallon of warm water.
Coffee cup stain remover	Moist salt.
Coffee pot stain	Vinegar.
Copper cleaner	Lemon juice and salt.
Decal remover	Soak in white vinegar.
Fertilizer	Compost and vermicompost.
Fiberglass stain remover	Baking soda paste.
Flea & tick repellent	Scatter pine needles, fennel, rye or rosemary on pet's bed.
Flies (insects)	Well-watered pot of basil.
Floor cleaner	1 cup vinegar and 2 gallons water.
Garbage disposal deodorizer	Use citrus rind or ice cubes.
Grease fire	Douse with baking soda.
Grease removal	Borax on damp cloth.
Hand cleaner for paint/grease	Baby oil.
Ink spot remover	Cold water and 1 tablespoon cream of tar-tar and 1 tablespoon lemon juice.
Insects on plants	Put soapy water on leaves, then rinse.
Laundry detergent	Basic household soap.
Linoleum floor cleaner	1 cup white vinegar and 2 gallons water.
Mildew remover	Equal parts vinegar and salt.
Mosquito repellent	Burn citronella candles. Citronella oil is a volatile oil obtained from the leaves and stem of the plant Cymbopogon winteratus or Cymbopogon nardus. Mosquitoes hate it.
Multi-Purpose Cleaner	Mix 1/2 cup ammonia, 1/3 cup vinegar and 1/4 cup baking soda in 1 gallon of warm water.

FOR THIS:	TRY THIS:
Nematode (parasitic worms) repellent	Plant marigolds.
Oil stain remover	White chalk rubbed into stain before laundering. Not always effective but definitely eco-friendly.
Paint–oil-based/stain/spray	Water-based, non-aerosol paints.
Paint brush softener	Hot vinegar.
Perspiration spot remover	Baking soda.
Pet odor remover	Cider vinegar.
Porcelain cleaner	Make paste from baking soda and water. Let set, rub clean and rinse.
Refrigerator deodorizer	Open box of baking soda.
Rug/carpet cleaner	Club soda.
Rust removal (clothing)	Lemon juice and salt plus sunlight.
Rusty bolt/nut removal	Carbonated beverage.
Scorch mark removal	Grated onion.
Scouring powder	Baking soda.
Shaving cream	Brush and shaving soap.
Slug and snail repellent	Onion and marigold plants. Many insects hate marigold.
Spot remover	Club soda, lemon juice or salt.
Upholstery spot removal	Club soda.
Water mark removal	Toothpaste.
Water softener	1/4 cup vinegar.
Wine stain removal	Salt.
Wood polish	3 parts olive oil and 1 part white vinegar; almond or olive oil (interior unvarnished wood only).

References
1. Green CT.org. *Fast Facts on Household Cleaners:* http://www.greenct.org/FAST FA~1.HTM
2. U.S. Environmental Protection Agency. *Sources of Indoor Air Pollution–Organic Gases (Volatile Organic Compounds–VOCs):* http://www.epa.gov/iaq/voc.html
3. Hazardous Substances Research Centers (sponsored by the U.S. Environmental Protection Agency [EPA], the Department of Energy, and the Department of Defense, and private contributors): http://www.hsrc.org/index.html
4. U.S. Centers for Disease Control: http://www.cdc.gov/

5. Ott WR, Roberts JW. Everyday exposure to toxic pollutants. *Scientific American;* Feb. 1998:86-91.
6. Green CT. *Other common household toxics:* http://es.epa.gov/techinfo/facts/safe-fs.html
7. U.S. Environmental Protection Agency. *Toxics Release Inventory:* http://www.epa.gov/tri/

Chapter 12
A Close Look at the Air We Breathe

There are two major areas to consider—outdoor air and indoor air. You are subject to whatever is in the outdoor air. Obviously, you will be less able to affect the quality of the outdoor air than the effects you can have on your own home environment. But you can still make a difference outdoors as a member of a growing, enlightened and concerned citizenry. Unless otherwise noted, the majority of the information that follows can be found in the Environmental Protection Agency's "Latest Findings on National Air Quality: 2001".[1]

At the center of the book where all the color graphics are located there several maps of the United States that are specific to air pollution (Plates 10 and 11). I regret that I did not have the time or resources before this printing to have maps of the world showing similar problems or for that matter separate maps showing all respiratory toxin links individually, but these maps will help to drive the point home well enough to start.

Pollution releases by state can be viewed in Figures 1-6 in chapter 8 (pages 62-64.

Outdoor Air Quality
Some countries—unfortunately, not the majority—are trying to clean up the air over their respective land masses. Keep in mind that air is blowing around the world twenty-four hours a day. If we were to create air pollution in my hometown of Detroit, Michigan, for example, that insult to the environment would be felt all over the planet. That is why every person, in every city, in every nation, needs to do their share.

Although the U.S. EPA has made real progress in improving outdoor air quality, this is only the beginning. Remember: I believe EPA is working hard and does want to do their duty for us, but they can only do what they are given the authority to do and the funds to do it with. I also believe there are good people in other agencies in various nations that have the same good intent and the same limitations as the U.S. EPA. The free oxidative and system stresses on your body are very serious despite some of the good work that has been done by these agencies. It is crucial that you remember that the effects of these stresses are far worse than the human body was designed to handle. We were designed to live on a pristine pollution-free planet. Advances in technology and science that have taken us beyond the simple lives of hunter-gatherers has created an imbalance that cannot be compensated for by the best diet or the best of intentions. This is why it is essential to take the proper antioxidant every day, modify your diet as discussed earlier and take action to improve the quality of the air in your home and workplace. We will look at some explanations and definitions. Then we'll look at the improvements in outdoor air quality since the 1970s. There actually has been progress.

The U.S. EPA started working on the air pollution problem in the 1970s. They started by identifying six common air pollutants—or "criteria"—for which it established National Ambient Air Quality Standards (NAAQS) under the Clean Air Act:
- ground-level ozone
- particulate matter
- carbon monoxide (CO)

- nitrogen dioxide (NO$_2$)
- sulfur dioxide (SO$_2$)
- lead

Ambient–or surrounding–air concentration levels are the key measure of air quality. These levels are based on the monitored amount (e.g., in units of micrograms per cubic meter [µg/m^3] or parts per million [ppm]) of a pollutant in the air.

Emissions levels are based on estimates and monitored measurements of the amount (e.g., in units of tons) of a pollutant released to the air from various sources, such as vehicles and factories. Some emissions travel far from their source to be deposited on distant land and water. Others dissipate over time and distance. The health-based standards (National Ambient Air Quality Standards) for criteria pollutants are based on concentration levels. The pollutant concentration to which a person is exposed is just one of the factors that determine if health effects occur, and their severity if they do occur.

At elevated ambient levels, these pollutants–both alone and in combination–are associated with adverse effects on human health and on the environment. Breathing those pollutants at harmful levels can result in respiratory problems, hospitalization for heart or lung disease, and even premature death. They can also harm aquatic life, vegetation and animals, as well as create haze and reduce visibility. In setting the national primary standards for each of the pollutants, the EPA intended to protect public health and the environment, as required by the Clean Air Act.

"What's That Stuff in the Air?"

Information on air quality trends for criteria air pollutants is based on actual measurements of pollutant concentrations in the ambient air at more than 5,000 monitoring sites across the country. The data from those readings support the EPA's key indicators for measuring outdoor air quality trends and determine which areas meet Clean Air Act standards.

Trends in criteria air pollutants, visibility, acid deposits and toxic air pollutants provide a picture of the nation's air quality. Our nation's air quality is generally improving, as measured by declining concentrations of criteria air pollutants. Acid deposit levels of sulfate are declining in the eastern U.S., the area most affected by deposition. Toxic air pollutants, though not as widely measured as criteria pollutants, also appear to be declining. Yet many challenges remain.

For most parts of the country, the average ambient levels of lead, carbon monoxide (CO), nitrogen dioxide (NO$_2$), and sulfur dioxide (SO$_2$) are lower than the standards. But many people live in areas of the country that do not always meet the health-based standards for certain pollutants, especially ozone and particulate matter. In fact, more than 133 million people lived in areas where monitored air quality in 2001 was unhealthy at times because of high levels of at least one criteria air pollutant. Consult the charts in chapter 8 figure 5 and 10 at the center of the book that show pollution by state and the maps that show pollution by county in the U.S. If you live in one of those areas that have unhealthy air quality, you need to take more than the minimum of antioxidant support daily. Review chapter ten on antioxidants if you are unsure. You can also go to the EPA Web site for updates, and often information on air quality is available locally.

Based on EPA's Air Quality Index (AQI) data, the percentage of days on which air quality exceeded a health standard dropped from almost 10 percent in 1988 to 3 percent in 2001.

The EPA has conducted an analysis of 260 metropolitan statistical areas (MSAs) for the 1990 to 1999 time period. This study shows that in 212 MSAs, the average ambient concentrations for at least one of the criteria pollutants had downward trends. In 57 MSAs, there were upward trends for at least one pollutant (with 34 of the 57 MSAs showing significant upward trends).

As a whole, the results of the study showed significant improvements in urban air quality over the past decade.

Ozone is not emitted directly into the air. It is formed by the reaction of volatile organic compounds (VOCs), nitrogen oxides (NOx) and other chemical compounds in the presence of heat and sunlight, particularly in hot summer weather. Chemicals such as those that contribute to formation of ozone are collectively known as ozone precursors.

Particulate matter is emitted directly into the air. It is also formed when emissions of NO_2, SO_2 and other gases react in the atmosphere. With decreases in emissions of VOCs and other ozone precursors, 8-hour ozone concentrations fell by 11 percent nationally between 1982 and 2001.

All regions experienced improvement in 8-hour ozone levels during the last 20 years except the North Central region, which stayed almost unchanged. However in 2001, more than 110 million people lived in counties with concentrations higher at times than the 8-hour standard for ozone. Southern California, the eastern U.S. and many major metropolitan areas experience continuing ozone problems.

Nowhere to Run

In 2001, some 73 million people lived in counties where monitored air quality at times exceeded the standard for fine particulate matter (PM2). The number of people living in counties with air quality levels that exceed the standards for ozone and PM signals continuing problems.

Pollution is impairing visibility in some of the nation's parks and other protected areas. In 1999, average visibility for the worst days in the East was approximately 15 miles.

In the West, average visibility for the worst days was approximately 50 miles in 1999. Particulate matter is the major contributor to reduced visibility in this region, which can obscure natural vistas. Without the effects of pollution, the natural visibility in the U.S. is approximately 47 to 93 miles in the East and 124 to 186 miles in the West. The higher relative humidity levels in the East result in lower natural visibility. Before pollution then the visibility was at least 2.48 times and perhaps as much as 3.72 times greater than today with pollution. Wouldn't it be wonderful if our grandchildren could see as far as our grandparents did in incredible clear skies? Our forbears as recently as 1930 had far better views of this beautiful land than we do. What will our grandchildren see? I believe we can reach that point again if we all work together at all levels as I have discussed throughout this book.

Indoor Air: You're in Control.
Do you experience any of these symptoms?
- Eye irritation
- Nose irritation
- Throat irritation

- Headaches
- Muscle twitching
- Tingling sensations
- Convulsions
- Dizziness
- Weakness
- Nausea
- Confusion
- Episodes of increased chest pain in people with heart disease
- Fatigue in otherwise healthy people
- Disorientation
- Malaise
- Increased occurrence of respiratory tract infections, such as bronchitis and pneumonia, especially in children
- Increased occurrence of ear infections; build-up of fluid in the middle ear, especially in children
- Increased severity and frequency of asthma episodes
- Decreased lung function
- Sneezing
- Watery eyes
- Coughing
- Shortness of breath
- Fever
- Digestive problems

If so, the air quality in your home or apartment may be a significant factor.

In this book, I have already provided information from scientific studies on toxins in your home. Many of those toxins are chemicals that also pollute your air. Remember our discussion of the personal toxic dust cloud? (Notice that this section relates directly to selected information presented in some previous chapters.)

When it comes to indoor air, most people don't give it much thought. If they can breathe and they are not in pain or dead, the air must be okay. I have warned repeatedly that how you feel in the 21st century is no longer an accurate gauge of your health. Many people have experienced what seems to be sudden disease without any warning. I believe that such problems can brew inside you for years while you are apparently symptom-free. Health effects from indoor air pollutants, as with many other toxins, may be experienced soon after exposure, but more probably, years later. Then it will often be too late.

Immediate effects may show up after a single exposure or repeated exposures. These effects might include irritation of the eyes, nose or throat; headaches; dizziness or fatigue. Such immediate effects will usually be short-term and treatable. Sometimes the treatment will simply consist of eliminating the person's exposure to the source of the pollution, if it can be correctly identified.

Symptoms of some diseases–including asthma, hypersensitivity pneumonitis and humidifier fever–may also show up soon after exposure to some indoor air pollutants. Hypersensitivity pneumonitis represents a group of respiratory diseases that cause inflammation of the lung (specifically granulomatous cells). Most forms of hypersensitivity pneumonitis are caused by the inhalation of organic dusts or molds. Humidity fever is a respiratory illness caused by exposure to toxins from micro-organisms found in wet or moist areas in humidifiers and air conditioners. This is also called air conditioner or ventilation fever.

The likelihood of immediate reactions to indoor air pollutants depends on several factors, including age and pre-existing medical conditions. Sometimes, whether a person reacts to a pollutant depends on individual sensitivity, which can vary tremendously. Some people become sensitized to biological pollutants after repeated exposures. It appears that some people can become sensitized to chemical pollutants as well.

Certain immediate effects are similar to those of colds or other viral diseases. Therefore, it is often difficult to determine if the symptoms are a result of exposure to indoor air pollution. It is important to pay attention to the time and place the symptoms occur. If symptoms fade when a person is away from the home and return when the person returns, an effort should be made to identify indoor air sources that may be possible causes. However, don't jump to conclusions here: The absence of obvious symptoms doesn't necessarily mean the air is clean. Some effects may be made worse by an inadequate supply of outdoor air or from the heating, cooling or humidity conditions prevalent in the home. Open your windows whenever weather permits.

How Much Pollution is Acceptable?
While pollutants commonly found in indoor air are responsible for many harmful effects, there is considerable uncertainty about what concentrations or periods of exposure are necessary to produce specific health problems. People also react differently to indoor air pollutant exposure depending on their age, genetics and relative level of health. Some health effects occur after exposure to the average pollutant concentrations found in homes, while others are the result of the higher concentrations that occur for short periods of time.

We know that many of these air pollutants cause illness and disease in humans even if we do not yet know all the details. More research is needed to better understand these reactions, and research takes money as well as a level of awareness that will cause research to be initiated. (More detailed information on potential health effects from particular indoor air pollutants can be obtained from the EPA.)

The threats to your health from air pollutants include:
- Household cleaners
- Household pesticides
- Environmental tobacco smoke (ETS)
- Biological contaminants
- Formaldehyde
- Lead
- Radon
- Outdoor air toxins that come indoors
- Dysfunctional or contaminated ventilation systems

Let's discuss these threats while bearing in mind the following four common-sense actions you can take:
1. Eliminate the source where possible.
   a. Refer to our discussion of toxins in carpeting, including pesticides and lead. I have already offered some natural, non-toxic recipes and substitutions for toxic household products of all types, from pesticides to cleaners to metal polishes. So there is no excuse for continuing to use unsafe chemicals for any of these purposes.

b. Sources that contain asbestos which are sealed or undamaged should be left alone. Notify your local office of the EPA to find out how to dispose of asbestos. You must be exposed to asbestos to be harmed by it. It is wise to avoid handling the asbestos until it can be disposed of properly.

c. Gas stoves, furnaces and kerosene-burning sources can be adjusted to decrease the amount of emissions.

2. Improve ventilation.

a. Diluting the concentration of toxins will help reduce the risk to some degree. Forcing the toxic air outside or into a filtration device will contribute significantly to the quality of air in your home.

b. Clean your ventilation system only if there is evidence it will benefit you. EPA has published a document called, "Should You Have the Air Ducts in Your Home Cleaned?" This document explains what air duct cleaning is and provides guidance to help consumers decide whether to have the service performed. You will also find helpful information for choosing a duct cleaner, determining if cleaning has been done properly, and guidelines to prevent contamination of air ducts.

c. Some diseases, like humidifier fever, are associated with exposure to toxins from micro-organisms that can grow in large building ventilation systems. However, these diseases can also be traced to micro-organisms that grow in home heating and cooling systems, as well as humidifiers. Children, elderly people and people with breathing problems, allergies and lung diseases are particularly susceptible to disease-causing biological agents in the indoor air.

d. Advanced designs of new homes are starting to feature mechanical systems that bring outdoor air into the home. Some of these designs include energy-efficient heat recovery ventilators (also known as air-to-air heat exchangers). For more information about air-to-air heat exchangers, contact the Conservation and Renewable Energy Inquiry and Referral Service (CAREIRS), PO Box 3048, Merrifield, VA 22116. You may also wish to get information from the U.S. Green Building Council at www.usgbc.org, especially if you are building a new home.

3. Get air cleaners for your home.

a. There are many types and sizes of air cleaners on the market, ranging from relatively inexpensive table-top models to sophisticated and expensive whole-house systems. Some air cleaners are highly effective at particle removal. Others, including most table-top models, are in some cases significantly less efficient. Unfortunately, air cleaners are generally not designed to remove gaseous pollutants. This brings us back to the topic of ventilation.

b. The effectiveness of an air cleaner depends on how well it collects pollutants from indoor air (expressed as a percentage efficiency rate) and how much air it draws through the cleaning or filtering element (expressed in cubic feet per minute). A very efficient collector with a low air-circulation rate will not be effective, nor will a cleaner with a high air-circulation rate but a less efficient collector. The long-term performance of any air cleaner depends on maintaining it according to the manufacturer's directions. Since they filter toxins, air cleaners get dirty quickly. Unless they are kept clean, they cannot help your indoor air quality.

c. Another important factor in determining the effectiveness of an air cleaner is the strength of the pollutant source. Table-top air cleaners in particular may not remove satisfactory amounts of pollutants from strong nearby sources. People sensitive to particular sources may find that air cleaners are helpful only if they use more powerful units or several units in one room, depending on the size of the room and the source of the toxin.

d. Houseplants have been shown to reduce levels of some chemicals in laboratory experiments. However, as I have already pointed out, studies have been narrowly focused. Speaking objectively, there is currently no evidence that a reasonable number of houseplants will remove significant quantities of pollutants in homes and offices. In fact, it is possible to make things worse if you over-water your houseplants. Overly damp soil may promote the growth of micro-organisms that can subsequently become a biological contaminant.

e. Unfortunately air cleaners do not seem to reduce levels of radon and its decay products. The effectiveness of these devices is uncertain because they only partially remove the radon decay products and do not diminish the amount of radon entering the home.

4. Take an antioxidant twice daily
As I continue–keep reminding you, you cannot eat enough "healthy" food to get sufficient antioxidant protection. In today's environment, not taking the best antioxidant available is the same as asking to become a victim of free radical disease (known to be caused by airborne toxins).

Control the problem at the source wherever possible.
The Radon Factor
The most common source of indoor radon (rn) is uranium in the soil or rock on which homes are built, and radon exists in places you would never imagine. As uranium naturally breaks down, it releases radon gas, a colorless, odorless and radioactive gas. Radon is yet another toxin that your senses cannot detect. Radon gas enters homes through dirt floors, cracks in concrete walls and floors, floor drains and sumps. When radon becomes trapped in buildings and concentrations build up indoors, exposure to radon becomes a health concern.

Any home may have a radon problem. This means new and old homes, well-sealed and drafty homes, and homes with or without basements. Sometimes radon enters the home through well water. In a small number of homes, the building materials can emit radon, too. However, building materials rarely cause radon problems by themselves.

Health Effects of Radon
The predominant health effect associated with exposure to elevated levels of radon is lung cancer. Research suggests that swallowing water with high radon levels may pose risks, too. However, these risks are believed to be much lower than those from breathing air that contains radon. Major health organizations including the Centers for Disease Control and Prevention,[2] the American Lung Association (ALA),[3] and the American Medical Association,[4] agree with estimates that radon causes thousands of preventable lung cancer deaths each year. In 2004, the EPA estimated that radon causes about 21,000 deaths due to lung cancer per year in the United States.[5] In reality, this number might range from 7,000 to 30,000 deaths per year. If you smoke and your home has high radon levels, your risk of lung cancer is especially high.

Reducing Exposure to Radon in Homes

- Measure levels of radon in your home. You can't see radon, but it's not hard to find out if you have a radon problem in your home. Testing is easy and should only take a little of your time. There are many kinds of inexpensive, do-it-yourself radon test kits you can get through the mail and from hardware stores and other retail stores. The EPA recommends that consumers use test kits that are state-certified or have met the requirements of some national radon proficiency program. Go to the EPA's Radon Web site for more information. You should call your state radon office to obtain a list of qualified contractors in your area. You may also contact either the National Environmental Health Association (NEHA) at www.neha.org or the National Radon Safety Board (NRSB) at www.nrsb.org for a list of proficient radon measurement and/or mitigation contractors.
- Treat radon-contaminated well water. Radon in water will be not a problem in homes served by most public water supplies, but it has been found in well water. If you've tested the air in your home and found a radon problem, and you have a well, contact a lab certified to measure radiation in water to have your water tested. Radon problems in water can be readily fixed. Call your state radon office or the EPA Drinking Water Hotline (800-426-4791) for more information.

Environmental Tobacco Smoke (ETS)

Environmental tobacco smoke (ETS) is the mixture of smoke that comes from the burning end of a cigarette, pipe or cigar, plus the smoke exhaled by the smoker. It is a complex mixture of over 4,000 compounds, more than 40 of which are known to cause cancer in humans or animals, and many of which are strong irritants. ETS is often referred to as "second-hand smoke" and exposure to ETS is often called "passive smoking."

In 1992, the EPA completed a major assessment of the respiratory health risks of ETS (Respiratory Health Effects of Passive Smoking: Lung Cancer and Other Disorders EPA/600/6-90/006F).[6] The report concludes that exposure to ETS is responsible for approximately 3,000 lung cancer deaths each year in non-smoking adults and impairs the respiratory health of hundreds of thousands of children.

Infants and young children whose parents smoke in their presence are at increased risk of lower respiratory tract infections (pneumonia and bronchitis) and are more likely to have symptoms of respiratory irritation like cough, excess phlegm and wheezing. The EPA estimates that passive smoking annually causes between 150,000 and 300,000 lower respiratory tract infections in infants and children under 18 months of age, resulting in between 7,500 and 15,000 hospitalizations each year. These children may also have a build-up of fluid in the middle ear, which can lead to ear infections. Older children who have been exposed to second-hand smoke may have slightly reduced lung function.

Asthmatic children are especially at risk. The EPA estimates that exposure to second-hand smoke increases the number of episodes and severity of symptoms in hundreds of thousands of asthmatic children and may cause thousands of non-asthmatic children to develop the disease each year. The EPA estimates that between 200,000 and one million asthmatic children have their condition made worse by exposure to second-hand smoke each year.

Exposure to second-hand smoke causes eye, nose and throat irritation. It may also affect the cardiovascular system, and some studies have linked exposure to second-hand smoke with the onset of chest pain. For publications about ETS, go to the Smoke-Free Homes Web site or the IAQ Publications page or contact EPA's Indoor Air Quality

Information Clearinghouse (IAQ INFO), (800) 438-4318 or (703) 356-4020.

Reduce Exposure to Environmental Tobacco Smoke.

- *Don't smoke at home or permit others to smoke in your home. Ask smokers to smoke outdoors.* The 1986 Surgeon General's report concluded that physical separation of smokers and non-smokers in a common air space, such as different rooms within the same house, may reduce–but not eliminate–non-smokers' exposure to environmental tobacco smoke.[7]

- *If smoking indoors cannot be avoided, increase ventilation in the area where smoking takes place.* Open windows or use exhaust fans. We have already discussed the importance of ventilation in reducing exposure to indoor air pollutants. Ventilation will also reduce but not eliminate exposure to environmental tobacco smoke. Because smoking produces such large amounts of pollutants, natural or mechanical ventilation techniques do not remove them from the air in your home as quickly as they build up. In addition, the large increases in ventilation it takes to significantly reduce exposure to environmental tobacco smoke can also increase energy usage and costs substantially. Common sense says the most effective way to reduce exposure to environmental tobacco smoke in the home is to eliminate smoking in the home.

- *Do not smoke if children are present, particularly infants and toddlers.* Children are particularly susceptible to the effects of passive smoking. Do not allow baby-sitters or others who work in your home to smoke indoors. Discourage others from smoking around children. Find out about the smoking policies of the day care center providers, schools and other caregivers for your children. If they have no current policy or their policy does not protect children from exposure to ETS, find a different caregiver. No excuses!

Biological Contaminants Abound

Biological contaminants include bacteria, molds, mildew, viruses, animal dander, cat saliva, house dust mites, cockroaches and pollen. In addition, the protein in urine from rats and mice is a potent allergen. When it dries, it can become airborne.

There are numerous sources of biological pollutants. Contaminated central air handling systems can become breeding grounds for mold, mildew and other sources of biological contaminants and can then distribute these contaminants through the home. (Remember that we spoke of cleaning the ventilations systems and your unit filters earlier.)

By controlling the relative humidity level in a home, the growth of some sources of biological pollutants can be minimized. As mentioned before, a relative humidity of 30-50 percent is generally recommended for homes. Standing water, water-damaged materials or wet surfaces also serve as a breeding ground for molds, mildews, bacteria and insects. House dust mites, the source of one of the most powerful biological allergens, grow in damp, warm environments. If you smell mildew, there is a problem. If you are in a hotel and you smell must or mildew from the ventilation system, change rooms or change hotels. Be sure to make the management aware of this situation.

Health Effects of Biological Contaminants

Some biological contaminants trigger allergic reactions, including hypersensitivity pneumonitis, allergic rhinitis and various types of asthma. Infectious illnesses, such as influenza, measles and chicken pox, are transmitted through the air. Molds and mildews release disease-causing toxins. Symptoms of health problems caused by biological pollutants include sneezing, watery eyes, coughing, shortness of breath, dizziness, lethargy, fever and digestive problems.

Allergic reactions occur only after repeated exposure to a specific biological allergen. That reaction might occur immediately upon re-exposure or after multiple exposures since you may become sensitized to it. *Immune support is of paramount importance in these cases.* **As a result, people who have noticed only mild allergic reactions, or no reactions at all, may suddenly find themselves very sensitive to particular allergens.**

Some diseases, such as humidifier fever, are associated with exposure to toxins from micro-organisms that can grow in large building ventilation systems. However, these diseases can also be traced to micro-organisms that grow in home heating and cooling systems and humidifiers. Children, elderly people and people with breathing problems, allergies and lung diseases are particularly susceptible to disease-causing biological agents in the indoor air.

Reduce Exposure to Biological Contaminants

- *Use exhaust fans that are vented to the outdoors in kitchens and bathrooms. Vent clothes dryers outdoors.* These actions can eliminate much of the moisture that builds up from everyday activities. There are exhaust fans on the market that produce little noise, an important consideration for some people. Another benefit to using kitchen and bathroom exhaust fans is that they can reduce levels of organic pollutants that vaporize from hot water used in showers and dishwashers.

- *Ventilate the attic and crawl spaces to prevent moisture build-up.* Keeping humidity levels in these areas below 50 percent can prevent water condensation on building materials.

- *If using cool mist or ultrasonic humidifiers, clean appliances according to manufacturer's instructions. Refill with fresh filtered water daily.* Since these humidifiers can become breeding grounds for biological contaminants, they have the potential to cause diseases such as hypersensitivity pneumonitis and humidifier fever. These diseases are serious, so don't be lazy about cleaning those units and changing the water daily. Evaporation trays in air conditioners, dehumidifiers and refrigerators should also be cleaned frequently for the same reasons.

- *Thoroughly clean and dry water-damaged carpets and building materials (within 24 hours if possible) or consider removal and replacement.* Water-damaged carpets and building materials can harbor mold and bacteria. It is very difficult to completely rid such materials of biological contaminants because they settle deep into the nap, the padding or even underneath the padding.
- *Keep your house clean. House dust mites, pollens, animal dander and other allergy-causing agents can be reduced, although not eliminated, through regular cleaning.* People allergic to these pollutants should use allergen-proof mattress encase-

ments. Wash bedding in hot (130° F) water. Avoid room furnishings that accumulate dust, especially if they cannot be washed in hot water. Allergic individuals should leave the house while it is being vacuumed since vacuuming can actually increase airborne levels of mite allergens and other biological contaminants. Using central vacuum systems that are vented to the outdoors or vacuums with high-efficiency filters may also be of help, as I mentioned earlier.

- *Take steps to minimize biological pollutants in basements.* Clean and disinfect the basement floor drain regularly. Do not finish a basement below ground level unless all water leaks are patched and outdoor ventilation and adequate heat to prevent condensation are provided. Operate a dehumidifier in the basement if needed to keep relative humidity levels (yes, you guessed it) between 30-50 percent. The U.S. Consumer Product Safety Commission and the American Lung Association can both provide more information on biological pollutants in your home.

Stoves, Heaters, Fireplaces and Chimneys

In addition to environmental tobacco smoke, other sources of combustion products are unvented kerosene and gas space heaters, woodstoves, fireplaces and gas stoves. The major pollutants released are carbon monoxide, nitrogen dioxide and particles. Unvented kerosene heaters may also generate acid aerosols.

Combustion gases and particles also come from chimneys and flues that have been improperly installed or maintained, plus cracked furnace heat exchangers. Pollutants from fireplaces and woodstoves with no dedicated outdoor air supply can be "back-drafted" from the chimney into the living space, particularly in weatherized homes.

Health Effects of Combustion Products

Carbon monoxide (CO) is a colorless, odorless gas that interferes with the delivery of oxygen throughout the body. At high concentrations, it can cause unconsciousness and death. Lower concentrations can cause a range of symptoms, from headaches, dizziness, weakness, nausea, confusion and disorientation to fatigue in healthy people. It can also cause episodes of increased chest pain in people with chronic heart disease. The symptoms of carbon monoxide poisoning are sometimes confused with the flu or food poisoning. Fetuses, infants, elderly people and people with anemia or a history of heart or respiratory disease can be especially sensitive to carbon monoxide exposures.

Nitrogen dioxide (NO_2) is yet another colorless, odorless gas. It irritates the mucous membranes in the eye, nose and throat and causes shortness of breath after exposure to high concentrations. There is evidence that high concentrations or continued exposure to low levels of nitrogen dioxide increase the risk of respiratory infection. There is also evidence from animal studies that repeated exposures to elevated nitrogen dioxide levels may lead or contribute to the development of lung disease, such as emphysema. People at particular risk from exposure to nitrogen dioxide include children and individuals with asthma and other respiratory diseases.

Particles, released when fuels are incompletely burned, can lodge in the lungs and irritate or damage lung tissue. A number of pollutants, including radon and benzo(a) pyrene–both of which can cause cancer–attach to small particles that are inhaled and then carried deep into the lung.

Reduce Exposure to Combustion Products in Homes

- *Take special precautions when operating fuel-burning unvented space heaters.* Consider potential effects of indoor air pollution if you use an unvented kerosene or gas space heater. Follow the manufacturer's directions, especially instructions about the proper fuel and keeping the heater properly adjusted. A persistently yellow-tipped flame is generally an indicator of maladjustment and increased pollutant emissions. When a space heater is being used, open a door from the room to the rest of the house from where the heater is located. Open a window slightly. Your best option is simply not to use unvented kerosene or gas space heaters.

- *Install and use exhaust fans over gas cooking stoves and ranges and keep the burners properly adjusted.* Using a stove hood with a fan vented to the outdoors greatly reduces exposure to pollutants during cooking. Improper adjustment, often indicated by a persistently yellow-tipped flame, can cause increased pollutant emissions. Ask your gas company to adjust the burner so that the flame tip will be blue. If you want to purchase a new gas stove or range, consider buying one with pilotless ignition since it will not have a pilot light burning continuously. Never use a gas stove to heat your home. And always make certain the flue in your gas fireplace is open when the fireplace is in use.

- *Keep woodstove emissions to a minimum. Choose properly sized new stoves that are certified as having met EPA emissions standards.* Make sure that doors in old woodstoves are tight-fitting. Use aged or cured (dried) wood only. Follow the manufacturer's directions for starting, stoking and putting out the fire in woodstoves. Chemicals are used to pressure-treat wood. Such wood should <u>never be burned indoors</u>. Some old gaskets in woodstove doors contain asbestos. When replacing old gaskets, refer to the instructions in the EPA booklet, *Asbestos in Your Home,* to avoid creating an asbestos problem. Newer gaskets are made of fiberglass. ·

I enjoy a wood fire as much as the next person. I believe the warmth and beauty of a wood fire has been ingrained into our genetic memory from our distant ancestors. Wood fire gives us a unique feeling of security and serenity. *But for a very long list of reasons, I urge you either not to have or to limit wood fires and follow the tips above.*

- *Have central air handling systems, including furnaces, flues and chimneys, inspected annually and promptly repair cracks or damaged parts.* Blocked, leaky or damaged chimneys or flues can release harmful combustion gases and particles, and possibly even fatal concentrations of carbon monoxide. Strictly follow all service and maintenance procedures recommended by the manufacturer, including directions that tell you how frequently to change the filter. If manufacturer's instructions are not readily available, change filters once every month or two during extended periods of use. Proper maintenance is important even for new furnaces because they can also corrode and leak combustion gases, including carbon monoxide.

About Household Products

Organic chemicals are now widely used as ingredients in household products. Paints, varnishes and wax all contain organic solvents, as do many cleaning, disinfecting, cosmetic, degreasing and hobby products. Fuels are composed of organic chemicals. All of these products can release organic compounds as you use them and, to some degree, even when they are stored.

The EPA's Total Exposure Assessment Methodology (TEAM) that I spoke of in an earlier chapter found levels of about a dozen common organic pollutants to be two to five times higher inside homes than outside, regardless of whether the homes were located in rural or highly industrial areas. Recall that other non-government studies that have studied indoor air pollution indicated 3-5 times (and even 10 times) more than outdoors. Additional TEAM studies indicate that while people are using products containing organic chemicals, they can expose themselves and others to very high pollutant levels. Elevated concentrations can persist in the air long after the activity is completed.

Health Effects of Household Chemicals

The extent to which organic chemicals cause health problems varies greatly, from those that are highly toxic to those with no known health effects. As with other pollutants, the extent and nature of any specific effect will depend on many factors, including level of exposure and length of time exposed. Eye and respiratory tract irritation, headaches, dizziness, visual disorders and memory impairment are among the immediate symptoms that some people have experienced soon after exposure to selected organics.

At present, not much is known about what health effects occur from the levels of organics usually found in homes. Many organic compounds are known to cause cancer in animals. In addition, some are suspected of causing cancer in humans.

- *Follow label instructions carefully.* Potentially hazardous products often (but not always) have warnings aimed at reducing exposure to the user. For example, if a label says to use the product in a well-ventilated area, go outdoors or to areas equipped with an exhaust fan. Otherwise, open up windows to provide the maximum amount of outdoor air possible.

- *Throw away partially full containers of old or unneeded chemicals.* Since gases can leak even from closed containers, this single step significantly lowers the concentrations of organic chemicals in your home. Be sure that materials you decide to keep are stored in well-ventilated areas safely out of reach of children. Do not simply toss these unwanted products in the garbage can. Find out if your local government or any organization in your community sponsors special days for the collection of toxic household wastes. If such days are available, use them to dispose of the unwanted containers safely. If no such collection days are available, take action in your community to get one started.

- *Keep exposure to emissions from products containing methylene chloride to a minimum.* Consumer products that contain methylene chloride include paint strippers, adhesive removers and aerosol spray paints. Methylene chloride is known to cause cancer in animals. Also, methylene chloride is converted to carbon monoxide in the body and can cause symptoms associated with exposure to carbon monoxide. Carefully read the labels containing health hazard information and cautions on the proper use of these products. Use products that contain methylene chloride outdoors when possible; use indoors only if the area is well ventilated.

- *Keep exposure to benzene to a minimum.* Benzene is a proven human carcinogen.

The main indoor sources of this chemical are environmental tobacco smoke, stored fuels and paint supplies, plus automobile emissions in attached garages. Benzene is found in all combustible engine fuels, from cars to jet airliners. To reduce benzene exposure, eliminate smoking in the home, provide maximum ventilation during painting and discard paint supplies and special fuels that will not be used immediately.

• *Keep exposure to perchloroethylene emissions from newly dry-cleaned materials to a minimum.* I hope you will agree that we thoroughly covered perchloroethylene (called Perc in the industry) in another chapter. But I am going to repeat it here, in case the reader likes to skip and scan rather than read the text in depth. Perc is, of course, something you must breathe in. Perchloroethylene is the chemical most widely used in dry cleaning. In laboratory studies, it has been shown to cause cancer in animals. People breathe low levels of this chemical both in homes where dry-cleaned goods are stored and as they wear dry-cleaned clothing. Dry cleaners recapture the Perc during the dry-cleaning process so they can save money by reusing it. They remove more of the chemical during the pressing and finishing processes.

Some dry cleaners, however, do not remove as much Perc as possible all of the time. Taking steps to minimize your exposure to this chemical is just common sense. If dry-cleaned goods have a strong chemical odor, do not accept them until they have been properly dried. If goods with a chemical odor are returned to you on subsequent visits, try a different dry cleaner. Some cleaners now provide what is called wet cleaning and do not use Perc. Inquire the next time you go. If possible, get a press-only service on your clothes unless cleaning is really necessary.

Understand Formaldehyde

Formaldehyde is a colorless, pungent-smelling gas that can cause watery eyes, burning sensations in the eyes and throat, nausea and difficulty in breathing in some humans exposed at elevated levels (above 0.1 parts per million). High concentrations may trigger attacks in people with asthma. There is evidence that some people can develop a sensitivity to formaldehyde. It has also been shown to cause cancer in animals and may cause cancer in humans.

Formaldehyde is widely used by industry to manufacture building materials and numerous household products. It is also a by-product of combustion and certain other natural processes. It is omnipresent in the modern world and extremely likely to be in your home and office.

Sources of formaldehyde in the home include building materials, smoking, household products and the use of unvented, fuel-burning appliances, like gas stoves or kerosene space heaters. Formaldehyde, by itself or in combination with other chemicals, serves a number of purposes in manufactured products. For example, it is used to add permanent-press qualities to clothing and draperies, as a component in glues and adhesives, and as a preservative in some paints and coating products.

In homes, the most significant sources of formaldehyde are likely to be pressed wood products made using adhesives that contain urea-formaldehyde (UF) resins. Pressed wood products made for indoor use include particleboard (used as subflooring and shelving and in cabinetry and furniture); hardwood plywood paneling (used for decorative wall coverings and in cabinets and furniture); and medium-density fiberboard (used for drawer fronts, cabinets and furniture tops). Medium-density fiberboard contains a higher resin-to-wood ratio than any other UF-pressed wood product and is generally recognized as being the highest formaldehyde-emitting pressed wood product.

Other pressed wood products, such as softwood plywood and flake- or oriented-strandboard, are produced for exterior construction use and contain the dark, red/black-colored phenol-formaldehyde (PF) resin. Although formaldehyde is present in both types of resins, pressed woods that contain PF resin generally emit formaldehyde at considerably lower rates than those containing UF resin.

Since 1985, the Department of Housing and Urban Development (HUD) has permitted only the use of plywood and particleboard that conform to specified formaldehyde emission limits in the construction of prefabricated and mobile homes. This is progress! But the government is protecting industry by allowing the chemical to be used at any level. In the past, some of these homes had elevated levels of formaldehyde because of the large amount of high-emitting pressed wood products used in construction and their relatively small interior space.

The rates at which products like pressed wood or textiles release formaldehyde can change. Formaldehyde emissions generally decrease as products age. When the products are new, high indoor temperatures or humidity can cause increased release of formaldehyde from these products. I have interviewed people who have purchased a new mobile home and complained of virtually all the known symptoms of high formaldehyde exposure. Sales people of mobile homes routinely recommend airing out the homes for up to two weeks before moving in. But formaldehyde is not just in mobile homes.

During the 1970s, many homeowners had urea-formaldehyde foam insulation (UFFI) installed in the wall cavities of their homes as an energy conservation measure. However, many of these homes were found to have relatively high indoor concentrations of formaldehyde soon after the UFFI installation. Few homes are now being insulated with this product. Studies show that formaldehyde emissions from UFFI decline over time. Therefore, homes in which UFFI was installed many years ago are unlikely to have high levels of formaldehyde now.

Reduce Exposure to Formaldehyde in Homes
Always ask about the formaldehyde content of pressed wood products, including building materials, cabinetry and furniture, before you purchase them.

If you experience adverse reactions to formaldehyde, you may want to avoid the use of pressed wood products and other formaldehyde-emitting goods. Even if you do not experience such reactions, you may wish to reduce your exposure as much as possible by purchasing exterior-grade products that emit less formaldehyde. You can get more information about formaldehyde content in consumer products by calling the EPA Toxic Substance Control Act (TSCA) assistance line (202-554-1404).

Some studies suggest that coating pressed wood products with polyurethane may reduce formaldehyde emissions for some period of time. To be effective, any such coating must cover all surfaces and edges and remain intact. Wear a mask while applying because the fumes are also toxic. If it smells toxic, it typically is.

Bearing this fact in mind, increase ventilation and carefully follow the manufacturer's instructions while applying these coatings. Some polyurethane coatings actually contain formaldehyde. Check the label contents before purchasing coating products to avoid buying products that contain formaldehyde. Maintain moderate temperature and humidity levels. The rate at which formaldehyde is released is accelerated by heat and may also depend somewhat on the humidity level. Therefore, the use of dehumidifiers and air conditioning to control humidity and maintain a moderate temperature can also help reduce formaldehyde emissions. Remember to drain and clean dehumidifier collection trays frequently so that they will not become a breeding ground for micro-organisms that can become biological contaminants.

Generally increasing the rate of ventilation in your home will greatly help in reducing formaldehyde levels.

Pesticides Can Bug You, Too

While I discussed pesticides at length earlier in this book, once again I know there are many who will simply skim through for areas of specific interest and not read the entire text thoroughly. Since inhaling pesticides presents a danger as well as exposure to skin going through your pores, it is appropriate to cover them here as well. (For the natural non-toxic replacements for dangerous pesticides, please refer to chapter 11.)

The products used most often are insecticides and disinfectants, which are also considered pesticides. One study suggests that 80 percent of most people's exposure to pesticides occurs indoors, and that measurable levels of up to a dozen pesticides have been found in the air inside homes.[8]

The amount of pesticides found in homes appears to be greater than can be explained by the amount of pesticides actually used in those households. Other possible sources include contaminated soil and dust that floats or is tracked in from outside and then deposited in carpets from our shoes. Carpets collect and then release the pesticides into the air again as we walk on the carpet. Stored pesticide containers may also leak pesticide vapors gradually. Pesticides used in and around the home include products to control insects (insecticides), termites (termiticides), rodents (rodenticides), fungi (fungicides) and microbes (disinfectants). They are sold as sprays, liquids, sticks, powders, crystals, balls and foggers.

In 1990, the American Association of Poison Control Centers reported that some 79,000 children were involved in common household pesticide poisonings or exposures. In households with children under five years old, almost one-half stored at least one pesticide product within reach of children.[9]

EPA registers pesticides for use and requires manufacturers to put information on the label about when and how to use the pesticide. It is important to remember that the "-cide" in pesticides means "to kill." This is deadly serious business–these products can be dangerous if not used properly and carefully.

In addition to the active ingredient, pesticides are made up of ingredients that are used to carry the active agent. These carrier agents are called "inerts" in pesticides when they are not toxic to the targeted pest. Nevertheless, some inerts are capable of causing health problems in humans. At least six inerts have been confirmed to cause illness in humans, and 94 others are suspected to be toxic as well. Up to 90% of some pesticide products are made up of these so-called inerts.

Health Effects from Pesticides

Both the active and inert ingredients in pesticides can be organic compounds. Therefore, both could add to the levels of airborne organics inside homes. Both types of ingredients can cause the effects discussed in this chapter. However, as with other household products, there is insufficient understanding at present about what pesticide concentrations are necessary to produce these effects. That doesn't mean we should not take precautions. It simply means we don't know how much poison is enough. To me, any amount of poison is too much, particularly as the effects of some of these chemicals are cumulative. You may be symptom-free for years before the onset of disease.

Exposure to high levels of cyclodiene pesticides has produced various symptoms, including headaches, dizziness, muscle twitching, weakness, tingling sensations and nausea. In addition, the EPA is concerned that cyclodienes might cause long-term damage to the liver and the central nervous system, as well as an increased risk of cancer. (Did you think you don't need supplemental support daily?)

There is no further sale or commercial use permitted for the following cyclodiene or related pesticides–chlordane, aldrin, dieldrin and heptachlor. However, heptachlor is still being used by utility companies to control fire ants in underground cable boxes.

Reduce Your Exposure to Pesticides in the Home
Use pesticides (if you must) in recommended amounts only because increasing the amount does not offer more protection against pests and can be harmful to you and your plants and pets. This recommendation by itself is reason enough to read this book!

• Ventilate the area well after pesticide use.

Mix or dilute pesticides outdoors or in a well-ventilated area and only in the amounts that are immediately needed. If possible, take plants and pets outside when applying pesticides to them.

Use non-chemical methods of pest control whenever possible. Since pesticides can be found far from the site of their original application, it is prudent to reduce the use of chemical pesticides outdoors as well as indoors. Depending on the site and pest to be controlled, one or more of the following steps may be effective:

• Use biological pesticides, such as *Bacillus thuringiensis,* for the control of gypsy moths; selection of disease-resistant plants; and frequent washing of indoor plants and pets.

• Termite damage can be reduced or prevented by making certain that wooden building materials do not come into direct contact with the soil and by storing firewood away from the home. By appropriately fertilizing, watering and aerating lawns, the need for chemical pesticide treatments of lawns can be dramatically reduced.

Don't forget that in Chapter 11, you have a number of natural, non-toxic pesticide recipes.

• *If you decide to use a pest control company, choose one carefully.*

Ask for an inspection of your home and get a written control program for evaluation before you sign any contract for work. The control program should list specific names of pests to be controlled and chemicals to be used. It should also reflect any of your safety concerns. Insist on a proven record of competence and customer satisfaction.

• *Dispose of unwanted pesticides safely.* If you have unused or partially used pesticide containers to get rid of, dispose of them according to the directions on the label or on special household hazardous waste collection days. If there are no such collection days in your community, work with others to organize them.

- *Keep exposure to moth repellents to a minimum.* One pesticide often found in the home is paradichlorobenzene, a commonly used active ingredient in moth repellents. This chemical has been proven to cause cancer in animals, and substantial scientific uncertainty exists over the effects, if any, of long-term human exposure to paradichlorobenzene. The EPA requires that products containing paradichlorobenzene bear warnings such as "avoid breathing vapors" to warn users of potential short-term toxic effects. Where possible, paradichlorobenzene, and items to be protected against moths, should be placed in trunks or other containers that can be stored in areas separately ventilated from the home, such as attics and detached garages.

Paradichlorobenzene is also the key active ingredient in many air fresheners. In fact, some labels for moth repellents recommend that these same products be used as air fresheners or deodorants. Proper ventilation and basic household cleanliness will go a long way toward preventing unpleasant odors. (What elected officials let that happen?) If it causes cancer to any mammal, we should not be using it as an air freshener.

It is irresponsible for any industry (in the name of profits) to put us at risk with an excuse like, "We are uncertain if it kills humans." Citrus and flowers and things that grow naturally on this planet provide wonderful, safe fragrances.

The EPA sponsors the **National Pesticide Telecommunications Network (NPTN)**, (800-858-PEST) to answer your questions about pesticides and to provide selected EPA publications on pesticides.

An Asbestos Primer

Asbestos becomes less of a problem every year, but it still exists, and you need to know about it. It is a mineral fiber that has been used commonly in a variety of building construction materials for insulation and as a fire-retardant. The EPA and CPSC have banned several asbestos products. Manufacturers have also voluntarily limited uses of asbestos. Today, asbestos is most commonly found in furnace insulation materials, asbestos shingles, millboard, textured paints and other coating materials, and floor tiles.

Elevated concentrations of airborne asbestos can occur after asbestos-containing materials are disturbed by cutting, sanding or other remodeling activities. Improper attempts to remove these materials can release asbestos fibers into the air in homes, increasing asbestos levels and endangering people living in those homes.

Health Effects of Asbestos

The most dangerous asbestos fibers are too small to be visible. After they are inhaled, they can remain and accumulate in the lungs. Asbestos can cause lung cancer, mesothelioma (a cancer of the chest and abdominal linings) and asbestosis (irreversible lung scarring that can be fatal). Symptoms of these diseases do not show up until many years after exposure began. Most people with asbestos-related diseases were exposed to elevated concentrations on the job. Some developed disease from exposure to clothing and equipment brought home from job sites.

Reduce Exposure to Asbestos in Homes

- *If you think your home may have asbestos, don't panic!* Usually, it is best to leave asbestos material that is in good condition alone. Material in good condition will not release asbestos fiber. There is no danger unless fibers are released and inhaled into the lungs.

- *Do not cut, rip, or sand asbestos-containing materials.* Leave undamaged materials alone and, to the extent possible, prevent them from being damaged, disturbed or touched. Periodically inspect these materials for damage or deterioration. Discard damaged or worn asbestos gloves, stovetop pads or ironing board covers.

Check with local health, environmental or other appropriate officials to find out about proper handling and disposal procedures.

If asbestos material is more than slightly damaged, or if you are going to make changes in your home that might disturb it, have a professional remove or repair it. Before you have your house remodeled, find out whether asbestos materials are present.

- *When you need to remove or clean up asbestos, use a professionally trained contractor.* Select a contractor only after careful discussion of the problems in your home. Learn the steps the contractor will take to clean up or remove these problems. Consider the option of sealing off the materials instead of removing them.

Call the EPA's TSCA assistance line at (202) 554-1404 to find out whether your state has a training and certification program for asbestos removal contractors and for information on EPA's asbestos programs. **(www.epa.gov/asbestos)**

Toxic Substances Control Act (TSCA) Hotline–Sponsored by the Office of Pollution Prevention and Toxics, the TSCA Hotline provides technical assistance and information about asbestos programs implemented under TSCA. These programs include the Asbestos School Hazard Abatement Act (ASHAA), the Asbestos Hazard Emergency Response Act (AHERA), and the Asbestos School Hazard Abatement Reauthorization Act (ASHARA). The Hotline provides copies of TSCA information, such as Federal Register notices and support documents, to requestors through its clearinghouse function.

E-mail address: **tsca-hotline@epa.gov**
Hours of service: 8:30 a.m.-5:00 p.m. (ET),
M-F Telephone: (202) 554-1404
TDD: (202) 554-0551
Fax: (202) 554-5603 (Fax available 24 hours a day)

Lead–Unhealthy Plus

Lead has long been recognized as a harmful environmental pollutant. In late 1991, the Secretary of the Department of Health and Human Services called lead the *"...number one environmental threat to the health of children in the United States."*

There are many ways in which humans are exposed to lead–through air, drinking water, food, contaminated soil, deteriorating paint and dust. Airborne lead enters the body when an individual breathes or swallows lead particles or dust once it has settled. Before we understood how harmful lead could be, it was freely used in paint, gasoline, water pipes and many other everyday products.

Old lead-based paint is the most significant source of lead exposure in the U.S. today. Harmful exposures to lead can be created when lead-based paint is improperly removed from surfaces by dry scraping, sanding or open-flame burning. High concentrations of airborne lead particles in homes can also result from lead dust from outdoor sources, including contaminated soil tracked inside and use of lead in certain indoor activities, such as soldering and stained-glass making.

Health Effects of Exposure to Lead

Lead can affect practically all systems within the body. At high levels, it can cause convulsions, coma and even death. Lower levels of lead can adversely affect the brain, central nervous system, blood cells and kidneys.

The effects of lead exposure on fetuses and young children can be severe. They include delays in physical and mental development, lower IQ levels, shortened attention spans and increased behavioral problems. Fetuses, infants and children are more vulnerable to lead exposure than adults since lead is more easily absorbed into growing bodies. The tissues of small children are more sensitive to the damaging effects of lead than those of adults. Children may have higher exposures since they are more likely to get lead dust on their hands and then put their fingers or other lead-contaminated objects into their mouths. Also, the presence of lead has been documented in the carpets of houses tested at random. Young children will naturally get higher exposure since they are close to the carpet most of the day.

Have your pediatrician test your child for lead exposure even if they seem healthy–particularly if they have delays in physical and mental development, lower IQ levels, shortened attention spans and increased behavioral problems. ADD and ADHD are not caused by Ritalin deficiencies. But, as you have already learned in this book, there are numerous toxins that can affect your child's attention span and behavior. If you see any of the above symptoms in your child, you should consider having them tested for the presence of toxins. To find out where to do this, call your doctor or local health clinic. For more information on health effects, get a copy of the Centers for Disease Control's Preventing Lead Poisoning in Young Children (October 1991).

Reduce Exposure to Lead

- *Keep areas where children play as dust-free and clean as possible.* Mop floors and wipe window ledges and chewable surfaces like cribs with a solution of powdered automatic dishwasher detergent in warm water. For this purpose, powdered dishwasher detergents are recommended because of their high content of phosphate. Most multipurpose cleaners will not remove lead from ordinary dust. Wash toys and stuffed animals regularly. Make sure that children wash their hands before meals, naptime and bedtime.

- *Reduce the risk from lead-based paint.* Most homes built before 1960 contain heavily leaded paint. Some homes built as recently as 1978 may also contain lead paint. This paint could be on window frames, walls, the outside of homes or other surfaces. Do not burn painted wood since it may contain lead.

- *Leave lead-based paint undisturbed if it is in good condition.* Do not sand or burn off paint that may contain lead. Lead paint in good condition is usually not a problem except in places where painted surfaces rub against each other and create dust (for example, opening a window).

- *Do not remove lead paint yourself.* Individuals have been poisoned by scraping or sanding lead paint because these activities generate large amounts of lead dust.

Consult your state health or housing department for suggestions on which private laboratories or public agencies may be able to help test your home for the presence of lead in paint. Home test kits cannot detect small amounts of lead under some conditions. Hire a person with special training for correcting lead paint problems to remove lead-based paint. Occupants, especially children and pregnant women, should leave the building until all work is finished and clean-up is done.

For additional information dealing with lead-based paint abatement contact the Department of Housing and Urban Development for the following two documents: *Comprehensive and Workable Plan for the Abatement of Lead-Based Paint in Privately Owned Housing: Report to Congress* (December 7, 1990) and *Lead-Based Paint: Interim Guidelines for Hazard Identification and Abatement in Public and Indian Housing* (September 1990).

- *Do not bring lead dust into the home.* If you work in construction, demolition, painting, with batteries, in a radiator repair shop or lead factory, or your hobby involves lead, you may unknowingly bring lead into your home on your hands or clothes. You may also be tracking in lead from soil around your home. Soil very close to homes may be contaminated from lead paint on the exterior of the building. Soil along roads and highways may be contaminated from years of exhaust fumes from cars and trucks that used leaded gas.

  Use doormats to wipe your feet before entering the home. If you work with lead in your job or a hobby, change clothes before you go home and wash these clothes separately. Encourage your children to play in sand and grassy areas instead of dirt, which sticks to fingers and toys. Try to keep your children from eating dirt, and make sure they wash their hands as soon as they come inside.

- *Find out about lead in drinking water.* Usually, most well and city water will not contain lead. Water usually picks up lead inside the home from household plumbing that has been made with lead materials. The only way to know if there is lead in drinking water is to have it tested. Contact the local health department or the water supplier to find out how to get the water tested. Send for the EPA pamphlet, Lead and Your Drinking Water. For more information about what you can do if you have lead in your drinking water, call EPA's Safe Drinking Water Hotline (800-426-4791).

- *Diet can help your kids fight lead.* A child who gets enough iron and calcium will absorb less lead. However, it is important to note that few children are iron-deficient. The leading cause of poisoning in children is iron poisoning from children's chewable vitamins, according to the Centers for Poison control. You may wish to seek a children's chewable that is iron-free since foods rich in iron include eggs, red meats and beans. Dairy products are high in calcium, not iron. Do not store food or liquid in lead crystal glassware or imported or old pottery. If you reuse old plastic bags to store or carry food, keep the printing on the outside of the bag.

References

1. U.S. Environmental Protection Agency. *Latest Findings on National Air Quality: 2001, Status and Trends,* EPA 454-K-02-001. Research Triangle Park, NC: U.S. Environmental Protection Agency, Office of Air Quality Planning and Standards, September 2002.
2. Centers for Disease Control. Churchill County (Fallon), Nevada Exposure Assessment. February 6, 2003: http://www.cdc.gov/nceh/clusters/Fallon/faq-radon.htm
3. American Lung Association. Search LungUSA. http://www.lungusa.org/site/apps/s/

content.asp?c=dvLUK9O0E&b=34706&content_id={3CEE8D57-6993-43A1-84AA-B908097E4650}

4. Stephenson J. Radon risk. *JAMA* 1998;279:818-b.
5. U.S. Environmental Protection Agency. January Was National Radon Month. http://www.epa.gov/radon/rnactionmonth.html
6. U.S. Environmental Protection Agency. *Fact sheet: Respiratory health effects of passive smoking.* EPA Document Number 43-F-93-003, January 1993.
7. U.S. Department of Health and Human Services. 1986 Surgeon general's report physical separation of smokers: The Health Consequences of Involuntary Smoking. A Report of the Surgeon General. U.S. Government Printing Office, Washington D.C., 1986.
8. U.S. Environmental Protection Agency. Sources of Indoor Air Pollution: Pesticides. http://www.epa.gov/iaq/pesticid.html
9. Litovitz TL, Bailey KM, Schmitz BF, et al. 1990 annual report of the American Association of Poison Control Centers National Data Collection System. *Am J Emerg Med.* 1991;9(5):461-509.

Chapter 13
Water Conservation—How You Can Make a Difference

It is urgently important that everyone become aware as soon as possible of the need to conserve water. So I am going to begin with some facts about water you probably didn't know.

All the water that exists today is the same amount as existed at the birth of this planet. Does that surprise you? Water simply recycles itself through evaporation and precipitation. If we pollute our water beyond our ability to clean it, we will eventually run out of clean water, and that will mean the end of all life on this planet.

Although approximately two-thirds of our planet is covered with water, only three percent of that is fresh water. Only one percent of all the water on this planet is available for human consumption, because the other two percent is locked up in the polar ice caps, according to the U.S. Environmental Protection Agency (EPA). Make no mistake; it is in fact possible to contaminate water beyond any method of treatment currently known so that it becomes forever unavailable for human consumption. In fact, we are already doing it. That is why this chapter is so critical.

We need to conserve the clean water, to try to keep from polluting water in general and to find new ways to reclaim toxic water. In most countries, people and governments aren't doing a very good job. We take water for granted in modern nations since we turn on the tap, and it magically always appears. But if we don't all act together, the day will come when that tap will be dry or what comes out of the tap might be liquid but not drinkable. Let me repeat if we do not all work together the day will come when there is no clean water left on planet Earth! Yes we have time, but not infinite time, so we need to start now.

Get Back to Basics
First, let's look at some quick water facts:
- 66 percent of a human being is water.
- 75 percent of the human brain is water.
- 76 percent of human muscle is water.
- 75 percent of a living tree is water. (Remember: Without trees, we would have no oxygen to breathe.)
- You could survive about a month without food, but only 5 to 7 days without water.
- On the average, every American uses about 160 gallons of water a day at a cost of 27 cents (EPA).
- Bottled water may cost up to 1000 times more than municipal water, but may not be as safe (EPA).
- Two-thirds of the water used in an average home is used in the bathroom.
- It takes about 39,000 gallons of water to produce the average domestic automobile, including tires (EPA).
- It is no longer safe for hikers and backpackers to drink water directly from remote streams (EPA).
- An acre of corn contributes more to humidity than a lake of the same size, but crops require huge amounts of water to grow.

Water Conservation Actions You Can Take Now

1. Don't allow water to run when brushing teeth or washing dishes.
- On the average, a person uses 2 gallons of water to brush his or her teeth each day, nearly 99% of which just runs down the drain never touching the toothbrush or your mouth. So open the tap to wet or rinse, then close the tap quickly. It could save countless millions of gallons if we all took this simple step. (Men, that goes for shaving too.)

2. Don't wash your cars or pets on a concrete surface.
- Washing you car on average uses up 20 to 30 gallons of water.
- Wash cars and pets over a grassy area, so that the water used will reduce the need for watering the area.
- Wash cars with a bucket instead of a hose, or go to a commercial car wash that recycles water.

3. Don't let the hose run unnecessarily when working outdoors.
- The average homeowner uses 240 gallons of water per half hour watering the lawn.
- Control the flow with a water nozzle.

4. Don't waste water by flushing tissues or hair down the toilet.
- This can eventually lead to clogs. Paper in water causes a pollution factor in and of itself.
- Save water and dispose of those things in a trash can.

5. Take short showers instead of baths.
- The average bath takes between 35 and 40 gallons. A five-minute shower, even without a water saver nozzle, will use up about 25 gallons–even less with a water saver. U.S. sailors and Marines know that "shipboard showers" can be done in two minutes or less. You don't have to do two-minute showers, but you don't need twenty-minute showers either.

6. If you live in the U.S., is your toilet a pre-1992 model? If so, you flush from 3 to 6 gallons every time you flush.
- Post-1992 toilets in the U.S. use only 1.6 gallons of water per flush. According to the EPA, a family of four can save up to 25,000 gallons of water a year by upgrading to a high-efficiency toilet. Replace your old toilets as soon as possible.

7. Washing dishes can use 10-15 gallons of water.
- If you can afford a dishwasher, shop for the model that conserves the most water and energy. Don't buy by brand name or aesthetics. Law regulates the energy facts displayed on the device, and you can depend on their accuracy.

8. Don't use extra rinse cycles on your dishwasher unless you absolutely have too.
- To save energy–not just water–don't use the high-energy drying cycle. Set the dishwasher to run before you go to bed and let dishes dry naturally overnight. That not only saves energy, but also saves you money.

9. Don't pour chemical products down the drain.
- You can help prevent pollution of drinking water sources by carefully disposing of

the chemical products you use in your home.

10. Don't over-fill at the gas pump or spill gasoline on the ground.
- One gallon of gasoline can contaminate approximately 750,000 gallons of water. That is enough water for 4,687 people to use in one day. Every ounce counts. That one-ounce of spilled gasoline could contaminate 5,859.4 gallons of water.

11. Stop Leaks.
- According to the EPA, a silent leak in a toilet, for example, in the most extreme scenario, can waste 500 gallons a day and cost $1,000 a year. All equipment or systems using water should be thoroughly checked for leaks.

12. Keep drinking water in the refrigerator instead of running the tap until the water gets cold.

13. Sweep sidewalks rather than hosing them off.

14. Change to water-efficient plumbing fixtures and appliances.

15. Replace Old Clothes Washers.
- A clothes washer is the second-largest water user in your home. Washers with EPA's Energy Star certification use 35-50 percent less water and 50 percent less energy per load.

16. Wash only full loads in dishwashers and clothes washers.

17. Plant the right plants.
- Consider xeriscaping, a technique for creating attractive gardens that use less water and are drought-resistant.

18. Provide only as much water as plants need.
- Automatic watering systems can be a home's biggest water user and can overwater greenery.
- Adjust systems monthly and consider purchasing electronic sensors to better control irrigation.
- Recycle water for plants before sending it down the drain.

Save a Buck and Help Save Our Planet
If you don't believe water conservation is important, perhaps saving money will capture your attention. The EPA found that across the country a typical family of four spends about $820 on water and sewer charges per year. Reducing water use can save money. EPA calculates that a typical family of four can save $210 per year by simply changing appliances and fixtures before taking any of the other steps I mention in this chapter. Can you find a use for an extra $200 per year?

There is no such thing as an insignificant effort when it comes to water conservation. One of the actions I strongly recommend is to get single-handled faucets throughout your home. Encourage the same to be done in all work places. Encourage your elected officials to do the same in all public places. The time it takes to adjust the temperature on two-handled faucets wastes gallons of clean water per use per person.

In public places, infrared sensor-controlled faucets are most ideal. Although we may sometimes find it annoying that there is a spilt-second delay, these can save countless millions of gallons that would otherwise needlessly and literally go down the drain.

Let's put your personal contribution in perspective. If only a 100 million people (about 1/3 of the U.S. population) each reduced just the waste from brushing their teeth, they could save a minimum of 150,000 million gallons of water a day. That is 54,750,000,000 gallons per year! That is worth repeating. Nearly fifty-five billion gallons a year can come from one little change. Yes, you can make a big difference for our planet. Every little bit counts. Everyone's efforts, no matter how small they may seem on an individual basis, counts!

Saving water also improves environmental quality by diverting less water to municipal uses and preserving more water for streamflow and aquatic systems. Less water use also means less energy demand, which translates to fewer pollutants from power plants.

Across the country, communities have successfully tightened their water-usage belts. New York City, Seattle and Boston have all reduced their water use by over 20 percent.

You can visit the EPA Web site for more information on saving water at home. Just go to *www.epa.gov/owm/water-efficiency/index.htm* and *www.energystar.gov/products/clotheswashers.* You can also take a virtual tour of a water-saver home at *www.h2house.org*

Can Water Filters Help?

Tests have shown that many bottled water companies (not all) simply sell tap water. Some tell you that on the label, some don't. Many people who buy bottled tap water are unaware of this fact because they just don't read the labels. Many are equally surprised to find that the standards for bottled water are no different than those for tap water.

When it comes to bottled water, three primary issues arise:
- General filtration of toxins, including chlorine, chlorinated hydrocarbons, trihalomethanes, pesticides, asbestos, particulate matter and heavy metals.
- Parasites, such as giardia and cryptosporidium, as well as bacteria.
- Pharmaceutical drugs.

The Compound-Combining Effect

Something you may not have thought is what I call the compound-combining effect. I introduced another new word above–"trihalomethanes." These are created when chlorine reacts with organic matter in the water. You may see it defined as reacting with decaying organic matter, but the fact is they can react with any organic matter. This group of organic halides contaminates as much as 90% of this country's drinking water. The four compounds–including chloroform (banned as an anesthetic in 1976)–are either known or suspected of causing cancer.

Trihalomethanes present one more reason to have a filter that at least removes chlorine. If you heat water that contains chlorine and then combine it with an organic–such as a refreshing, healthful herbal tea–the result typically has five times the level of trihalomethanes. So your cup of healthful tea, combined with hot water that contains chlorine, could actually be increasing your risk of cancer.

According to an article in *U.S. News & World Report* (July 29, 1991 issue) titled "Is Your Water Safe?–The Dangerous State of Your Water," drinking chlorinated water may as much as double the risk of bladder cancer, which struck about 40,000 people a year at that time.

> **"Cancer risk among people drinking chlorinated water is 93% higher than among those whose water does not contain chlorine."**
> –U.S. Council of Environmental Quality

General filtration

The public's understanding of water filtration systems is poor at best. I cannot speak for every government, but the U.S. government has enacted two important rules when it comes to rating water systems. First, nothing is 100%, so the best you will ever see in the U.S. is 99.9% in any category. In the case of some toxins, 98% is as good as it gets, but that percentage is still hugely beneficial as compared to the alternative. Second, it is not legal to say "removes toxins" because that implies that 100% is removed. Therefore, companies must say reduce rather than remove.

At the time of writing this book, I have yet to see any purification system of any type or at any price that has been third-party tested and confirmed to remove 100% (or even 99.9%) of all known pollutants as well as all the pharmaceutical drugs discussed in chapter 7. Yes, many companies make all manner of claims, and I receive many contacts from people who have been convinced by marketing materials cleverly disguised as scientific proof that convinces them to spend incredible amounts of money on filtration systems and devices. However, I feel it's important to repeat: At this moment, I have yet to see a system that removes 100% of the toxins and pharmaceuticals, as validated by third-party testing.

I need to make this point clear for everyone. Nobody at the time of publishing has tested for everything, and perhaps nobody ever will. It is not as straight-forward as you might imagine. Remember: There are more than 75,000 synthetics plus countless volatile organics and thousands of pharmaceutical drugs.

With this point in mind, one must make a leap of faith based on the data available. If the filter in question removes 98% or more of any toxin in a given category, it is likely that it will do the same for other toxins in the same category. So you should look for the longest and toughest list of toxins you can find for each product you research. Also look for that list to have been certified by a third-party lab or government agency. Currently, that is the best you can do.

Let's be clear about pharmaceuticals in your water

The idea that we all take virtually every known drug every time we drink water is pretty darn scary. As mentioned in Chapter 7, thus far in all communities tested, many categories of the drugs present (though not all) are not screened. There are thousands of drugs, and most water filtration companies don't even realize that there are drugs present in our drinking water. So, of course, they don't test for them.

Lets take this one mind-boggling step further: Since drugs have been detected in the drinking water of more than 100 cities, it is safe to assume they are widespread. But since tests have not revealed all known drugs, it is possible that certain drugs that combine create a totally new compound as yet unknown. So just what would we be testing for? That's the compound-combining effect. The thought of all the endless combinations and compounds that could theoretically result from combinations is beyond comprehension! Objectively speaking there is never likely to anything out there that is third party certified to remove all toxins.

Once again, it is not that there is not a system that could remove pharmaceuticals–I believe there probably is such a system. In fact, I am currently testing an organically based technology that I am hopeful will filter many drugs commonly found in drinking water. However, it is my duty to be objective, and there is a distinct difference between desire or belief and proven fact.

I do not have the time or resources to research every water filter made, so I don't want to leave you with the impression that I have personally checked them all. I will keep searching, and you should too. I am simply imparting what I have gleaned so far regarding water filtration. Every water filtration system claims to be the best, so be careful look for the third party certifications in all the areas mentioned above. Since education is what I do, it wouldn't hurt to educate you a bit on the types of filtration systems to help you make your choice.

Types of water filtration systems

- Sedimentation
- Carbon
- Hybrid Carbon
- Enhanced Hybrid Carbon
- Reverse Osmosis (RO)
- Distillation

Sedimentation is the most common and least expensive filter. It is primarily designed to remove large particulate matter like dirt and other particles from well water. By the way, well water has all the same contaminants as tap water, according to testing around the world. If toxins are going to be at the north and south poles, they are also likely to be everywhere in between. Some sedimentation filters do more than that, but not much more.

Carbon filters are well-advertised, so they are familiar. They are typically made of charcoal-based activated carbon and/or coconut shell-based activated carbon and are effective at reducing chlorine, some organics, some solvents, some pesticides and some heavy metals. Unfortunately, they don't reduce enough of the toxins, but they are certainly better than sedimentation or no filter at all.

Hybrid Carbon filters are made on the same principle, but are typically more expensive and more efficient than standard carbon filters. The basic filter upon which the hybrid is built is made from charcoal-based activated carbon and coconut shell-based activated carbon, but also has a porous plastic that is non-leaching (some plastics leach dangerous phthalates). This makes it adsorbent for specific contaminants like arsenic as well as fluoride-effective. This is another step up for filters and offers huge health benefits. Also, like its less sophisticated brother, the standard carbon filter, it reduces chlorine, some organics, some solvents, some pesticides and some heavy metals.

Enhanced Hybrid Carbon or Hybrid Carbon Plus

This type has all the basics and benefits of the Hybrid Carbon, but it is, as the name implies, enhanced. This type provides broad-spectrum reduction of contaminants, reducing all organics, all solvents, all pesticides, and heavy metals that have been tested for thus far.

It also has special enhancement media to produce what is typically referred to as "wetter water." Wetter water? Yes, that's what it is. The enhancement media has several benefits: First, it induces negative ions, causing a temporary realignment or restructuring of molecules so that it absorbs faster or hydrates better. It would be like having a lot of people trying to shove through a doorway at once–some will squeeze through here and there; or having all the people line up in an orderly single file to pass through more quickly and efficiently. Wetter water also helps you absorb nutrients more efficiently. The last (but, as the saying goes, not least) of the benefits is detoxification. For many, this type of filter can significantly reduce the symptoms of detoxification while increasing the efficiency of detoxification.

Reverse osmosis (RO) is very well-known, but not everyone understands it. To make RO as simple as possible, try to picture a tube with water in it sealed at both ends. The tube is made of a material that has such fine pores that the clean molecules squeeze through while unwanted material continues through the system. RO is more complicated than that, but this isn't a water filtration textbook!

RO water is very pure, but there is one big drawback. Water should be neutral or balanced. It should be 0 on the water stability index. Your body was designed to drink it that way. Well water or very hard water has a +stability index and that isn't good, but RO has a –stability index, and that is far worse. Some scientists refer to RO as "highly aggressive" water. It has nothing in it anymore that's not natural, but can actually dissolve things as a result. That certainly isn't advisable over the long term. I know those who have paid big bucks for an RO unit or those who sell them will be angry with me and want to set me straight, but these are the findings, and that's the way it is. Water needs to be neutral to be fully healthful.

Distillation offers the highest purity, but is extremely negative since it involves turning water into steam and then letting it condense back to water again. Rain water is nature's method of distillation. In fact, rain water is nature's way of cleansing our air. Water evaporated from heat goes into the atmosphere and returns again as rain or snow.

When water is distilled artificially, it changes in such a way that it attracts minerals–both the beneficial ones and the harmful ones. That is why distilled water is often recommended for detoxification, since its molecules actually attract and help remove certain unhealthful minerals. Over time, however, this could rob you of vitally healthful minerals. I had many patients when I was in practice who tested for deficiencies of healthful minerals because of long-term use of distilled water. This factor represents a very serious drawback.

	Water Stability Index	
+Stability	0 Neutral & natural	-Stability
Dissolves solids such as metals at extreme +	Healthful	Deposits solids such as minerals at extreme -

And now–you want to know which type of filter I use, don't you? I use an enhanced hybrid carbon filter. This method has many benefits without any drawbacks. Having said that, I have probably made an enemy of everyone who makes or sells anything other than an enhanced hybrid carbon filter. *Oh boy, just what I need–more enemies…*

I wouldn't blame the RO makers and sales people for wanting to come after me and take me down, as they say. But, my friends, I am simply doing the best I can to give you the best, most objective analysis I can for your benefit (certainly not mine). If the RO companies come up with data that is better than what I have represented, then by all means go for it. I want all companies to prosper as long as they are doing what's best for you! I would be almost 100% certain that none of the RO companies believe there is any problem with negative stability water. But if the stability is negative enough, *over time it can actually dissolve even steal.* Advocates of RO may argue that the water isn't in your body long enough to do any harm and it is extremely pure, so RO is the best.

And yes, the Water Stability Index is far more complex than this and leaves room for interpretation, but this is not a book about that specifically, and I need to educate all at every level.

My advice is to take your time, and shop wisely. If all you can afford is a $15 low-grade standard carbon filter, it is still hundreds of percent better than just plain tap water. Do what you can, but do something. You don't taste most of the chemicals in water that can cause cancer, nervous system disorders, infertility, behavioral disorders and immune disorders–but rest assured, they are there.

Okay! I have presented you with the basic facts in very simple terms to help you make your own best decision when you shop for a filtration unit.

How to Survive on a Toxic Planet

on a

Toxic Planet

SECTION 3

My
Journey

Dr. Steve Nugent

Chapter 14
Nothing Traditional

What follows in this chapter is <u>very</u> personal–so personal, in fact, that to the last moment before publication, I agonized over writing it and hesitated to add it to this book. I could have done without this chapter altogether. One of my most trusted business advisors said, "Don't write any of this since it detracts from the book. Let people form their own opinions about you from your work alone."

However, my *most trusted* advisor in life (as well as my best friend) urged me to tell all. She explained that my readers and critics need to know who I am and how I have arrived at this point in my life. I have spent more than half my life with that trusted friend, who also happens to be my beautiful wife, Wendy. Although my guts were twisted into knots while writing this chapter, over the years I have learned to trust her, and she is rarely wrong. So here is my non-traditional story. I hope it will help you understand me and understand my motivations in writing this book and doing the work I do.

* * * * *

How often I have said to myself, Why me God? Why did I have to take such a stressful path? My life has been nothing if not interesting. My life has always been nontraditional. I always find myself as the man in the middle, neither right nor left <u>attempting</u> to be the objective voice in a world of subjectivity. I have never enjoyed the comforts of being part of the mainstream. When someone says what do you do for a living, there is no short, simple answer. When someone says what college did you go to I have to ask them "for which degree program?" and then when I name some of the colleges I have attended to Americans (with the exception of one), I have to give lengthy explanations because only one of them had a football team, and the average American knows only of the famous schools of the Ivy league or those whose athletic programs (not always the best academics) get them on the news. So, instead of going through the following information in person 100,000 times, I have decided to put it in writing, and when someone asks, I will simply say, "Read my book."

I wish I would have had the privilege of attending Harvard, or Yale or one of the other world- renowned Ivy League schools, but financially that simply wasn't possible. I so often lament that I couldn't have taken a traditional "normal" path in education and career, but I also know that I had to take this path, because it has positively affected the lives of hundreds of thousand of people around the world, which will become millions in the future and that would have never had happened had I followed the easy, traditional path. Like the lesson from the movie called "It's A Wonderful Life" we all affect so many people in ways we often could never imagine.

I have always been obsessed with accumulating knowledge. My personal library is impressive to most everyone who sees it with shelves going all the way to my study's 12-foot ceilings, spanning the width of my nearly 18-foot walls. I am interested in a very wide range of nontraditional (even exotic) knowledge, as well as a few traditional areas of study, but health and human nutrition have been at the top of my list for a very long time.

Non-Traditional Pathways
My interest in human nutrition goes way back to the early seventies. I was looking for

a career path that did not exist at that time in the United States. So I began to take college courses without real direction initially–not especially unusual for a young person. I started on my Associates degree in the early seventies before I volunteered for the U.S. Marines (USMC). While in the Marines, I decided to take advantage of something called the Tuition Assistance Program that paid 75% of my college costs while I was on active duty, but did not take away from my GI Bill benefits.

I guess I have been in a hurry all my life, and my education was no different. I couldn't waste time and wait until I completed my military service to finish school, and the financial assistance from the USMC was too good to pass up. While I was stationed at Camp Pendleton I enrolled at National University (NU) in San Diego California, (I later attended several other of their campuses too). No, NU doesn't have a football team, but they do did have a very good soccer team and they are a *fully accredited* college. They had flexible class schedules evenings and weekends to help any working adult and that was particularly appealing to an active-duty Marine who wanted to further his education. I didn't have the luxury of just taking a few years off for school.

Periodically someone who thinks every college degree program is 4 years long attempts to figure my age by my degrees. Sorry, not all degree programs are four years long and besides I rarely do anything the traditional way. I am still grateful to the forward thinkers at National University for allowing me to accelerate my studies, taking a chance on me. I petitioned for, and was granted, permission to take a class schedule that was between 1 1/2 and 2 times faster than normal with a class load that simply wasn't done. The condition was that my grade point average never dropped below a B (3.0 out of possible 4.0). If it did I would be put back on a regular class load just like all the other students. The administration had no idea how tenaciously I will work towards a goal. I did better than keep a B average, and that surprised most everyone.

Regretfully, as that portion of my youth slipped by, I knew I was never to have the experience the traditional college campus and college life had to offer. I will probably always envy those who have had that experience. I did not have parents who could afford to help me–my father died when I was only 9, which left my mom to raise me on a secretary's small salary, barely enough to support herself. So, I needed to get my education the best way I could.

While taking that often-double class load, I distinguished myself as a Marine according to the citations from my commanding officers, and I also managed to graduate with top honors (*summa cum laude*) from my bachelors degree program even with that heavy class load. I was a newly wed with a young stepdaughter. They suffered by having very little of my time and attention, a trend which would continue I regret to say. So in the course of approximately five grueling years in the classroom, I completed my first three degrees. It would have been easy enough to apply for a traditional medical school at that time, but that didn't feel right to me inside. I didn't know why then, but after more than half a century of life and many tribulations, it is now clear. I had no idea at the time how that decision would change my life and many thousands of lives in the future.

Had I pursued the traditional path and become a medical doctor, my indoctrination would have been greatly different. I would have embarked on a path that would likely have never given me orientation or access to the study of non-traditional things that now are slowly but certainly being demanded by patients everywhere. I know my personality. Once I believe in something, I am unshakable and will fight for those beliefs to the last. *What if* I had been taught that drugs and surgery were the only way? Would I be one of the strongest critics against nutritional therapies today? The answer is likely yes. My life would have been so much easier, I would not have spent the last 25-plus years fighting against the ignorance of the so-called conventional wisdoms, I would not have been attacked from all corners. Why did I make that decision?

My Choice–Naturopathy

With my associates, bachelors and masters degrees in hand, I still did not have the knowledge I wanted or needed. So I continued my search. While working on my first doctorate (in psychology), I became more interested in the biochemistry of behavior than the counseling aspect. After all, brain chemistry is a result of vitamins, minerals, amino acids, glyconutrients and various co-factors not drugs. As I wrote in a 1996 newsletter, "No psychological disorder is caused by a drug deficiency." My mentor at the time explained to me that the only field that seemed to even remotely teach what I was interested in was something I had never heard of called *naturopathy*. What, you might ask, is that?

In the broadest and the original sense, naturopathy is the therapeutic use of things provided by nature, just as the name implies. The first health professionals, whether they were tribal shamans or Hippocrates himself, were all naturopaths. Every medicine and modality they used was from nature. It is ironic that allopaths (medical doctors)–even those who are staunchly opposed to natural therapies–had traditionally taken an oath created by a naturopath. To me, the most important words of that oath are, "Do no harm." Yes, the man revered as the Father of Medicine was a naturopath!

Scientifically validated natural therapies do no harm, while unexpected effects from properly prescribed (not from doctor error) drugs are the fourth-leading cause of death in most modern nations. Naturopathy is, in fact, the oldest of health professions. Yet it is still not universally accepted or standardized, nor is it a unified profession. Unfortunately, not all naturopaths are friends, nor is there one standard theory of practice within the profession as a whole. The level of scientific training among those who practice naturopathy also varies widely. Some naturopaths in some regions literally have no scientific training at all whereas some have equal levels of scientific training to medical doctors. Some rare naturopaths have even higher levels of scientific training.

At the time I decided to pursue naturopathy all those years ago, there were no big-name accredited schools and no government regulations regarding naturopathy in any nation. Naturopaths were thought of as quaint and folksy at best, but certainly not as doctors. So I had to piece-meal my education to fit what I thought could prepare me best to serve others. I had no idea where that particular fork in the road would lead me.

I pursued a doctor of naturopathic medicine (NMD) degree at Clayton University (CU), named for Clayton, Missouri, located near St Louis, which struggled to stay open (due to low enrollments) and ultimately closed. My choice of CU has been and I suspect will be criticized all my life by those who wish to discredit my work, but the quality of the course work was good enough to have their classes accepted in transfer by at least three different, regionally accredited colleges and earned them the U.S. Department of Education (USDE) pre-accredited status code 3IC. (By the way, the concept of regional accreditation seems to be unique to the U.S.) CU had to close their doors forever due to lack of funding before they could go further with the accreditation process. I received an excellent basic knowledge in all things traditionally naturopathic, but I needed more. What was missing was an understanding of how humans adapted to their environments–why certain genetic groups do better with one food than another, one climate than another, or one altitude than another. That is the study of biological anthropology.

Maize and Blue

So I enrolled in a special degree program at the University of Michigan's Dearborn campus (UMD), one of three University of Michigan campuses that existed at that time. All were University of Michigan—just different campus locations. I chose UM Dearborn rather than the more renowned UM Ann Arbor since Dearborn was the only campus I could find then that would let me design my own graduate degree program without wasting time on obligatory course work that would have no bearing on my career goals. Now, of course, it is common for progressive universities to work with students to arrange similar programs.

At that time, UMD offered something called the Professional Development Degree program, or PDD. They required that a student already have an undergrad degree before being admitted to this degree program. I designed a program that gave me much of what I felt I needed to complete the holistic health care picture, biological anthropology, biological psychology and traditional nutrition science.

Why traditional nutrition science? Because I needed to understand the other side, why universities taught that diet alone could make and keep you well, when naturopathy taught the opposite? I have taken many courses just to see the other side—all part of my being an objective thinker.

Although I was working very long hours in my clinic, my radio show and my public speaking engagements, as well as on my international newsletter and updating and publishing my doctors desk reference, I managed to complete this graduate program at University of Michigan with top honors as well. Any Michigan alumni will tell you that's no easy task under any circumstances. Yes, I bleed maize and blue (the school colors), as we Michigan alumni say. Oh, and by the way—the University of Michigan has the rare distinction of not only having great athletic teams, but always being rated in the top ten academically in the US. In fact, it is most often in the top five. The UMD campus was rated as one of America's top commuter campuses in America when I attended, and I suspect it is still rated very high.

In between those things listed and subsequent to them as well, I have taken many courses from various schools, plus two other non-traditional degree programs which I do not list in my biography. Yes—a total of 8 degrees. Please don't strain yourself doing the math—remember, I said "non-traditional."

Take Your Best Shots!

Now why do I spend the time on this topic? It is because I have been attacked by some of the most vicious critics you could ever imagine. I could write a book on the attacks I have suffered, and this book will surely cause an increase in those attacks. The first edition of this book has already increased my troubles and this second edition is greatly expanded so I expect things to intensify for me as a result. The critics' aim is to discredit my work because they fear it threatens their incomes and in most cases it challenges the knowledge upon which their status or reputations are built.

I strive for objectivity and that as I have said is not easy. So, many times through my research I have found that things I wanted to believe simply weren't correct. Scientific objectivity must win out regardless of ones desires or philosophies.

My critics cannot find fault in the science I present, so they attack my rather non-traditional path. It is amazing the lengths someone will go to protect their incomes or status. I was a pioneer. I did not have a paved road to follow; I had to pave it myself as I went.

Oh–how much simpler life would have been…

The entire printing of my first edition of this book sold out in less than six weeks with no advertising or publicity. I was both pleased and surprised by its success but now I am finding that I am getting negative input from some environmentalists who have read it and who think I am not extreme enough. *Gees…* Those environmentalists think I have not hit what they feel to be the most important issues. There a just a few who want me to stop trying to be balanced with my presentation and join with them on an all out assault against certain politicians or industries.

My goal is to convince everyone at every part of the political spectrum that we need to begin to take care of ourselves and our planet in ways they may not have previously imagined. If my presentation is not balanced and properly substantiated the critics will be able to discredit this work. I need to say at this point that I have respect for anyone who is willing to fight for what they believe in even if I disagree with them. But this is the path I must follow. Some people tend to turn off the mainstream population so much that the word Environmentalist is an immediate negative to millions of people who do not understand the Earth's delicate balance and what we can and must do for all life on this planet. And because they are turned off they will not spend the time and effort to learn how each person can play a critical role in the future of our world. Everyone needs to know the problems and the solutions so my approach will not change regardless of the criticism I receive.

I have also begun to receive attacks from various industries and commercial concerns that fear this book may hurt their earnings if the public finds out how big the problem is and acts on my recommendations.

Oh boy…

Not every attack has been vicious–some have just been interesting. After the first edition of this book was published, I had an interesting encounter. I gave a lecture at which an elected official (whose name I shall withhold) was in attendance (there have been three such occurrences, by the way, since the first edition was published). This politician was very angry with me, or, as they say in some circles, "vein-popping angry." He believed I was implying that all politicians are corrupt, and that is why our world is such a mess. I never said or implied that, however, and it certainly doesn't say that in my first edition or in this edition. Where did he get that idea? Was he feeling guilty?

I asked him, *"Sir, are you one of those corrupt politicians who accepts money from industry to cover up their messes or cares only about being re-elected rather than fulfilling your responsibility to your constituents?"* Of course, he replied angrily that he wasn't, and that was why he was mad at me. I then said, *"It was never my intention to offend anyone, and I have said nothing like what you have implied. But regardless of what you think you heard, I would suggest to you that you now have a great opportunity to be the first among your colleagues to take action. To introduce your peers to this information and to really make a difference for those who trusted you enough to elect you, I would be pleased… no, thrilled…to help you in any way I could to achieve that end."* I gave him my card and have never heard from him since. The other two politicians have not contacted me either. *Hmmm…*

Changing our environment is only part of the health care picture. And it is our abuse of the environment and the creation of a whole new world of toxins that has created the necessity of blending personal healthcare with environmental actions. That is the most unique aspect of this book. I was among the first to use the term "complementary med-icine" many years ago because it is my belief that we must all work together on this vital-ly important mission for health. Natural therapies that have been scientifically validated, as you have learned in this book, definitely complement traditional medical therapies, par-ticularly in the areas where pharmaceutical medicine alone simply can't save your life. I want you to think back in previous chapters to the strong positive data regarding nutri-tionals and cancers, as well as other diseases in this book. Remember what I always teach…"Nutrients are fuel not drugs or medicines. No nutrient cures the body. The body is designed to repair, regenerate, protect and heal itself, but it can only do that if it has the natural tools or fuel it needs to do the jobs it was designed to do. The body is the real miracle."

After I had been struggling in practice for a few years, I found out that there was a pro-fessional group for naturopaths and they claimed they were trying to get standardization and even licensing for naturopaths. I knew of no other similar group at the time. What I did not know was how much misery my involvement in naturopathic politics was going to cause me. According to some, naturopathy started in the US more than 100 years ago. But in reality, it is as old as the first natural remedy, going back many millennia. There are still records surviving today of disease protocols more than 5,000 years old that are made from all-natural substances. That's naturopathy.

Today there are actually three naturopathic groups, but only two major ones in the US. The oldest of these groups is no longer very active. Unfortunately members of the three groups don't always get along with each other. Few people know that all of the health-care professions went through a similar struggle before becoming standardized profes-sions.

This bitter fight goes back nearly thirty years and just like many wars in human history it was started and has been perpetuated through misinformation by a few which has resulted in irrational fear by the majority. It is (unfortunately) natural for most human beings to want to destroy what they fear. All naturopaths in fact all complementary med-icine practitioners should ultimately have the same goal and that is help people with their health through safe nontoxic means. But power struggles between the groups and yes even within the groups has created animosities that we may not be able to overcome in my lifetime. *That saddens me more than I can say.*

I was President of the second oldest and at that time the largest group in the Western Hemisphere for natural health care practitioners. I say at that time because I have not had any involvement in naturopathic politics since 1997 and I have no idea what the status is of any of the groups today. I served as President only three years of my four-year term when it became painfully clear that I would not be able to get the various factions to sit down and talk. I could not convince anyone from the third group to trust me enough to even have a telephone conversation and I could not keep the more volatile members of my own group from continuing their war against the third group, which fueled the mis-trust of course. Since I was president of the second group members of the third group simply had knee jerk reactions and without doing any objective research assumed I was leading or at least encouraging the attacks on them from some of the more radical mem-bers of my group. This never was the case, but I never had a chance to talk with their members rationally, so I quickly became their prime target.

It was Mostly About Philosophy

The group I was President of believed philosophically that naturopaths should only do those modalities that were non invasive and definitely non-toxic. We were of the belief that naturopathy was complementary to allopathic medicine not a replacement for it. Of course not even all the members of my group were united on that.

The third and newest group however had some members who openly advertised themselves as superior to medical doctors. *Antagonizing the medical profession seemed very counter productive to me.* The third group basically was looking for licensing to do just about anything an MD would do with the exception that drugs prescribed would have to be naturally based rather than synthetic. And of course not everyone in that group was in complete agreement with that philosophy either.

There were unfortunately members on both sides who were absolutely certain that their philosophies where the only correct ones. And they were (and some of them still are) willing to do almost anything to win. Court cases between the two groups go back to the seventies. If you isolate the first letter of the three words **We Are Right** it spells **WAR**.

I believe that the ideal doctor of the future is in fact one who is trained in both allopathic and naturopathic science. I would love to see licensing for naturopaths by class according to levels of scientific training. There are hundreds of thousands of people now who would I believe support me politically for the good of all and I would be delighted to be able to help all natural practitioners achieve their rightful place, if I could ever get all the factions to communicate with each other. My door is open.

One of the rumors spread among the third group about me was that my lectures where only about naturopathic politics and my goal was to discredit their group and their affiliates where ever I went. I have had people following my lectures since the eighties who will attest that I have never I repeat never once in any of my lectures in any country discussed naturopathic politics. The theme of this book has been the theme of my lectures since the early eighties. My detractors although I have attempted to invite them to my talks would never attend.

The other problem I have had from some of the more militant members of the third group is their knee jerk reactions to advertisements I did not create. You see naturopaths have been struggling for legitimacy in the health care community for a long time so arguments over credentials and competency seem to never end. I do not now and have never in the past advertised one of my lectures. I always lecture for a host upon invitation and it has always been that way. Some of the layman who have hosted me in various cites over the years have made some pretty colorful advertisements about me to promote a lecture which of course they have a strong financial stake in. Ultimately much stronger than mine because I get paid even if nobody attends. I had a sweet well meaning individual in Vancouver British Columbia for example create and distribute flyers before I arrived to lecture there that listed me as a brain surgeon from the Mayo Clinic. Gees...

By the time I arrived one day prior to the event the *"stuff"* had already hit the fan as the saying goes. The leader of the Canadian naturopaths in the province at that time acting on misinformation from some of the leaders of the third US naturopathic group combined with this clearly false information on a flyer I did not create, caused him to launch and obsessive campaign against me. He was obsessive and irrational he worked hard to intimidate the media and every TV and radio station in the city except one canceled the scheduled interviews that my host (not I) had arranged. He even tried to force my hotel to throw me out on the street. Yes, that's absolutely true. He tried to convince the Royal

Canadian Mounted Police (RCMP) to arrest me and of course they politely told him they had no reason to do so. There were even threatening notes left under my hotel room door. Yes it sounds crazy but it is absolutely true.

Imagine being in my position trying to figure out just what was going on? I never saw the flyer until after my talk and couldn't figure out what all the craziness was about. This has happened to me many times over the years this is just one example and not the most extreme one by the way. My host was near a nervous breakdown because of the calls he received almost hourly for many days prior to my arrival trying to intimidate him into canceling the lecture. He had rented the Vancouver convention center and that's a big investment. This naturopath convinced at least some of his members that I must be stopped from speaking at all cost and they came to the door of the center to intimidate attendees to not buy a ticket for the lecture. I attempted to contact this naturopath through mutual contacts and asked to meet with him but he refused to communicate with me by any method. Remember this man never met me and refused to have any contact with me yet devoted all his energy to my ruin. I have had to deal with this for years and there is no end in sight.

Two RCMP officers did attend my lecture, but not to arrest me. They came to hear about the latest facts on the environment and their health and what they could do about it. That's what I do after all. They both told me the lecture was great and they suggested I file charges against the Canadian naturopath who made my visit to Vancouver so miserable. One Canadian government official made the same suggestion, but I did not take action against him. By the way, we had more than 2,000 in attendance at the lecture despite all the trouble, so I believe I was meant to be there.

I have always found Canadians to be unusually polite, gracious people. In fact, I am so honored to say that in 1997 the Mayor of Edmonton Alberta Canada made me an honorary citizen after I had lectured to a near capacity crowd at their state of the art convention center. I am very proud and very honored because I have always been extremely fond of Canadians starting when I was a young boy growing up in Detroit only minutes by car from Windsor Canada. This is not about Canadians, but I use this example because Canadians are so nice as a culture that it is really hard to believe that this could happen.

So, very often before I arrive in a town local naturopaths affiliated with that third group have already launched all out campaigns against me. I tell you this so that if you attempt to talk with one of these individuals about this book you are likely to hear all manner of negatives about me from someone who has never met me and has no factual information about me and of course hasn't read this book. That is why I am telling far more than any author would ever tell unless he or she was writing an autobiography. This is who I am. Take it or leave it. My mission is to inform and educate as many people as I can on the dangers to human health from toxins, inadequate nutrition and to the survival of our planet no more and no less. I will not be dissuaded by anyone in that mission.

If my detractors would only take the time to find out who I am and what I do they would learn that I don't have horns or a tail and it is my deepest desire as I have said throughout this book that we must work together for the common good. Those who would harm life on this planet either knowingly or unknowingly for their own greed or power are my only enemies, and they should be yours too.

Another Difficult Choice
So many people think a person can only have one direction one interest or even only

one talent, so those people tend to be puzzled when they get bits and pieces of my history and try to piece it together. So, to add a little more confusion to my history, I have always been torn between my love of being a communicator, public speaker, teacher, and radio and television host, and my need to help people with their health, one-on-one. Recently I have realized that it is my ability in public speaking that has probably swayed more people to complementary medicine than anything I could ever have done in private practice. (*I'll never get a Pulitzer Prize for my writing!*)

I spent my last two years in the Marines as a broadcaster. Yes, each service has a handful of their own people for radio and television broadcasting as well as film making in addition to print journalism. I was trained as a broadcast information specialist at the Defense Information School (DINFOS) at Fort Benjamin Harrison in Indiana. In order to get this coveted training I had to extend my enlistment an extra nine months, which is why my term of voluntary enlistment was not four years like everyone else's. While I was awaiting my rigorous official training at DINFOS I was getting on the job training and was technically eligible to enter the international competition for the coveted Thomas Jefferson Award for military broadcasters. All of the seasoned broadcasters at the station laughed at me. They all entered the competition every year and never came close to wining, and I hadn't even been through school yet so why should I bother? I am not easily dissuaded from any goal so I did enter and I won the Thomas Jefferson Award (second place). I subsequently (after DINFOS) won top Marine Corps awards for radio broadcasting two years in a row. Yes, I love broadcasting! It comes very natural to me. So when you hear me on a tape or CD, yes, that really is me—not a paid professional announcer, and that really is my voice and yes that was my voice before DINFOS.

After the Marines, I continued my education and began to develop my career path as a nutritional consultant and health educator. In Michigan, there were no regulations for naturopaths—in fact, the word did not even exist in Michigan law. It was a real struggle to support my family and continue my education while also trying to develop my career, but an opportunity came up with my second love (broadcasting) that I simply couldn't pass up.

With my excellent training and considerable experience as a broadcaster in the Marines, I landed a job as a weekend and substitute talk show host for WXYZ radio in Detroit, which at that time was part of the American Broadcasting Company (ABC) Talk Radio network. Detroit was then the seventh-largest radio market in the United Sates. Even I was surprised by the popularity of my show, particularly when the station manager informed me that I was rated number one in my timeslot.

ABC finally sold WXYZ, and I had the great honor of doing the sign off broadcast of one of America's oldest radio stations. With my last broadcast a great part of American radio history came to an end. After that I worked on WPON (for many years) in Detroit (one health show per week) to keep my skills sharp. I also worked for WGPR in Detroit as a co-host for their morning news and talk show, which only took a few <u>very</u> early morning hours each day from my schedule.

I reached many thousands because of my experience on these shows. I have also been a guest on many shows throughout the United States, and in other countries as well. Not to mention the more than 100,000 people (at the time of this printing) I have reached through my lectures—many of them doctors of every discipline. My tapes, CD's and DVD's have reached even more people. Just one of the many tapes I produced sold over 400,000 copies in only three months just through word-of-mouth—no advertising at all. My audiences, I am happy to say, have always been strong and loyal.

Renewed Inspiration

I have also been blessed in that I have been able to help many tens of thousands with their health. I was in private practice for many years and had patients come from all over the world to my clinic. Most that came had been told they were at death's door and had little hope. My clinic was nicknamed "the last chance clinic" by my patients and colleagues. I have been personally responsible for saving many lives that I am aware of, and many more saved indirectly as a result of my lectures, my "Desk Reference for Applied Clinical Nutrition" (used by doctors), my tapes and my writings. I stopped publishing updates to my Desk reference in 96 but I may update it and bring it back due to demand.

In addition, I do regular teleconferences around the world. I was invited to participate on a conference call just before I started to write this last chapter of this book. The call I just spoke of reminded me of an old TV show, "This is Your Life." There were listeners from six countries on this call, numbering many thousands of people. One caller after another talked about how they wouldn't be alive today if it weren't for the information I provided them. It always helps me emotionally when I get the chance to hear overwhelming joy from people who are now well–people who at one time had little or no hope of being well. When I hear those most dramatic cases of those who had a death sentence from major medical centers but are still alive, well…it warms my heart and my soul and drives me on through all the adversity.

Learning From Personal Experience

The cases I have dealt with in my career have been extreme and exotic, and that could make a book in itself. My own family has suffered because, according to my wife, God had to force me to find answers for all the others who had no hope with those same afflictions. Wendy has a deep faith that has kept her strong, even when she faced her own and, later, our son's mortality.

Maybe her faith is so strong because she has actually visited to the other side. Does that sound crazy? Well, Wendy was clinically dead–not once, but twice!–back in 1986. She had a pulmonary embolism (PE) after what should have been a routine gallbladder surgery in 1986. She had no symptoms (a theme I have discussed ever since) prior to the sudden and extreme pain that put her into the ER. The first surgery didn't go well, she had a second operation, and then died again from another PE. From this experience, I learned an enormous amount of information about liver and gallbladder, PE's and the circulatory system after that–far above and beyond what is typically understood by the average doctor. And I'll be darned if I didn't get a veritable parade of people who needed help in those areas immediately following Wendy's near-death experiences.

In my wife's case she had the second operation because things went wrong from the first one. Forty–yes, forty!–doctors consulted on her case, and not one could figure it out. I tenaciously researched her case myself. Our son was only two at the time, and Wendy was much too young to die! *I found the answer*, and she is here today to try and keep me on the right path. I have helped so many people avoid surgeries, but I would not have completed that extra study had it not been for my wife's experience, I simply would have continued comfortably with what I had been taught in school as most doctors do. My non-traditional path forced (and continues to force) me to find unorthodox answers. I don't permit myself to stop just because there is no convenient, orthodox answer.

When my son, Danny, was nine, he was bitten by a mosquito that gave him viral encephalitis–a swelling in the brain due to the viral infection and extreme fever. It was a couple of days later that he went into a grand mal seizure.

When we rushed him to the hospital, they told us *it was not if he was going to die–just a question of when.* They said he would not survive the night, but if he did get past that hurdle, he would have permanent brain damage according to the neurologist (one of the best in Michigan at the time). After Danny had spent many weeks in the hospital, he was released with a grim future. *It was my turn now to help him.*

I already knew more than the average practitioner about nutrition and brain chemistry because of my highly unusual educational path, which definitely came in handy, but his "impossible" case forced me to do research outside of the customary box again.

The neurologist said Danny's brain damage affected his memory centers (the hippocampus, in this case), motor centers and cognitive function and was permanent. The first assessment was that he would never have the IQ of higher than a five-year-old, but that assessment improved over time. The brain damage was extensive. He was also expected to be an epileptic for the rest of his life due to damage in the hippocampus. Motor function, coordination and short-term memory were real and serious issues we had to work on, and I refused to accept that my son would never improve. This neurologist was an expert in what he was trained in, but he had no idea what dietary supplements could do! After all, the human body is the most miraculous creation, designed to heal itself. But it can only accomplish this miracle if provided with the appropriate fuel.

I gave Danny a series of nutritional therapies, and my wife prayed constantly. She never left his side, spending twenty-four hours a day in the hospital. One day, his short-term memory returned (despite the expert opinions), and his communications skills, which before the encephalitis were always ahead of his peers. His motor skills started to return to a normal level as well.

My son had multiple grand mal seizures everyday–some documented to last for hours. The only way to manage the seizures was with a drug called Dilantin (no other antiepileptic would work for him). All of my knowledge and research up to that time could not find a natural response to his seizures, which were occurring because of the damage in the hippocampus.

Then a very persistent representative of a nutritional company (one among many, I might add) started coming to my clinic and would not leave me alone until I agreed to look at the science behind a new class of nutritional products called *glyconutrients*. He is a giant of a man, and at the time I thought he was also a giant pain! I will always be grateful to him for changing the course of my life, as well as the lives of all those people who have thanked me for their health or even their lives since he introduced me to glyconutritionals. We owe him our gratitude for that too.

The science was clear that it couldn't hurt my son, and there was enough evidence even then to indicate that it might be the key to his full recovery. Over the course of the next year-and-a-half, I was able to gradually lower his dose of Dilantin until he needed none at all while he was taking glyconutrients. My son had extremely abnormal EEG's (brain wave scans), and each month they would check to see if he had made any progress.

After several months using this new nutritional technology, his EEGs were NORMAL! His doctor was so impressed that he started to send me his patients that he could not seem to help any further with conventional treatment. Now <u>that</u> is *complementary medicine*!

Since then, Danny has had no Dilantin and no seizures all these years later. As I write this text, my son is now twenty! Every loving parent brags about their kids, but objective testing shows my son's IQ is not only above that of a five-year-old, but is exceptional for any adult. In fact at the age of 20, he had already filed patents on his first two inventions!

Complementary therapies such as glyconutrients can make a world of difference where there would otherwise be no hope. This was not a placebo effect that my son experienced, he did not have a clue what was being done, and it wasn't isolated since countless numbers of my patients have also benefited strongly from glyconutrients–so much so that I made the decision to quit the security of my practice that I had fought so hard to build in order to tell the world about this new technology. I did not realize it at the time, but this decision was the beginning of even greater problems for me.

Is There a Bull's-Eye on Me?

When I began to strongly speak out for the newly discovered glyconutritional complex in 1996, the attacks against me reached a new level of fury. Some naturopaths as well as other practitioners feared that glyconutritionals would put them out of business. Even many from my own group turned against me since glyconutritionals were so effective that many other supplements were simply no longer necessary, and most naturopaths must also sell supplements to make a living in most states.

No matter what the attacks were against me, I kept up that fight because *this is information the public must know and the medical community must accept for the good of everyone,* as you have learned in this book.

I could have shown natural practitioners how to be successful–I did it the hard way, but I learned from my mistakes. In my last few years in practice, I had a patient waiting list never less than a year long. I had patients who came to see me literally from all over the world, including some who had to bring translators. I had medical doctors who not only wanted to work with me but also wanted to work for me in my clinic to both learn from me and enjoy that monetary success I created.

Before I was introduced to glyconutritionals, I had a strong and positive relationship with more than twenty nutritional companies, and I was one of the most sought-after speakers for their products. My lectures were fully objective, and my hosts allowed me to say for example, "Well, this company has 50 great products that I will train you on, but they also have two marginal ones, so I'll recommend a different company for those two". No company objected to my mentioning other companies in my talks because the doctors trusted that I would always give them a truthful, fully objective analysis and recommendation without sales pitches and no nonsense. That made the doctors stronger advocates of any products I recommended and was a huge benefit to any company I endorsed. None of those companies had anything truly revolutionary–simply better or worse quality of the same things everyone else had.

Then I began to talk about the importance of glyconutrients. That was revolutionary, and it did threaten many companies. At that point, I didn't have to burn my bridges since most (not all) the company reps burnt them for me. I suddenly found myself being attacked by reps of many different nutrition companies. Two companies continued a positive relationship with me and interestingly those were the two that had the best quality products and they new it. It is easy to be confident when you know you are right. Those who attacked me couldn't really find scientific fault with my presentations so they resorted to the kind of character assassination that persists to this day.

A Different Tactic

Some companies thought they could buy me. So, the temptations began. I have been offered very exciting positions and contracts with nutritional companies that didn't make glyconutritionals–companies that thought maybe if they had me, they could defeat this glyconutritional menace. How does 1% of all sales of all products of all types in a world-wide company sound? Wow! How about a three-year, $5 million contract and a position as Chief of Science with full control over product research and development? Full control over product research and development would be a dream come true, far more tempting than money. Would you be tempted?

Well…yes, I admit I did think about that last offer, but not for very long.

The path I have chosen will probably not allow me to be rich or have an easy life, but my rewards on this path cannot be measured in dollars.

My path to this point has been anything but traditional. My life could have been smooth and easy, but I believe we all have purpose in this life and that I have been direct-ed onto this unconventional path. Only on this strange path would I have been forced to learn things that would not have been taught to me in any medical school, university nutrition science department or even the best naturopathic college.

So in those quiet moments, I say to Him, "Okay, God. I understand what you want me to do, but why does it have to be so stressful?"

However, as I have learned in life, change only comes with necessity and frequently adversity. Usually change only happens under stressful situations, so I must walk on a non-traditional path…

I did not make the decision to write this book lightly. I think you can understand after reading the powerful information presented in this book that it will most likely bring me more controversy and emotional stress than I have ever experienced in my life. But this is a story that must be told. It must be told boldly and in simple terms. The public, all gov-ernments, the healthcare professions and industry must be moved to action. Our lives and the life of this planet are literally at stake. We all must work together!

Chapter 15
FINAL THOUGHTS

Yes, there is hope. There is hope to reclaim our environment. The City of Cleveland, Ohio proved that when they transformed their river, which was little more than a mucky sewer for the area, into a viable body of water. The river had been so polluted it had actually caught fire! Rivers aren't supposed to burn. Another sterling example is when Federal, state and local agencies worked to bring back Lake Erie from what was essentially a lifeless cesspool, dangerous to human and animal life, into a lake that can now be enjoyed by all. Lake Erie being one of the five Great Lakes covers 9,910 sq mi (25,700 sq km). It is more of an inland sea than a lake. That was a gigantic undertaking. But it proved it could be done!

When agencies like the U.S. EPA have the proper funding for research and the authority for enforcement of environmental laws, they have proven that they can significantly reduce the levels of air pollution. The potential to reclaim our planet and to ensure that this magnificent world will be here for all future generations to enjoy is very real. The opposite outcome unfortunately is just as real.

You have learned a huge volume of information in this book. Much of this is data you did not know. Some of it is data you wish you didn't know. But not knowing this information won't protect you from the dangers in our world that lead to disease, suffering and death. In most cases, this suffering is needless. You can make a difference. You now know what to do.

You know what to do to improve the health of your home and your workplace. You know what to do to work for political reform. And you know what to do in terms of diet.

Many of the changes can be made with the recipes and replacements given in this book, plus various actions you now know how to take for yourself and your family.

You know that no matter how much healthy food you eat, it cannot provide you with enough nutrition to protect you from the oxidative stress and other chemical stresses on your immune system, nervous system and reproductive system. Our bodies were designed to live in a pristine environment that no longer exists. They are not designed to cope with the stresses of today's world without considerable assistance. That assistance must come from scientifically validated dietary supplements that have been proven to give you the best known antioxidant and immune support. Dietary supplements are simply no longer a luxury–they are now a necessity. Your routine each day and the budget you put aside for groceries must include supplements. You can't eat enough groceries to give the protection these supplements can provide.

Beware my friends, there are those who either cannot face the realities in this book or those whose incomes or egos are threatened by this book. They will stop at nothing to keep you from knowing the truth and taking the actions necessary to preserve our environment.

I have already been attacked after the first edition of this book, and I expect it will get worse for me, but I would hasten to point out that not one of those attacks was objectively based. My work stands on its own–the science in this book is too strong for any reasonable person to ignore. Do not let those people dissuade you

from doing what must be done for our planet and our future generations.

There is much to be concerned about and much for us to do, but there is also great hope if we all act together. The choice is yours. Do what needs to be done and become a part of the solution, or do nothing and continue to be part of the problem. Do you choose to take care of yourself and your loved ones as directed in this book? Or do you choose suffering, disease and premature death from oxidative stress?

What would you choose for the children of Earth as yet unborn? A beautiful blue planet or a lifeless, toxic rock orbiting in the infinite vacuum of space?

You can make a difference...the choice is yours.

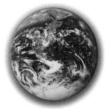

INDEX